"*The Awakened Therapist* is a visionary exploration, shedding light on often overlooked aspects of therapist consciousness and energetic attunement within the healing process. Through a transpersonal gestalt perspective, Harmony Kwiker offers invaluable insights and practical guidance for therapists, illustrating how heightened awareness shapes the therapeutic encounter."

Katie Asmus, MA, LPC, BMP, founder of
The Somatic Nature Therapy Institute

"*The Awakened Therapist* is a must-read for new and seasoned therapists who want to discover the healing potential of transpersonal gestalt counseling. Harmony has offered us a clear and profound account of how to stay connected to our true nature as we hold space for clients."

Arielle Schwartz, PhD, author of *The Post-Traumatic Growth Guidebook* and *The Complex PTSD Workbook*

"*The Awakened Therapist* is a marvelous book that shows therapists how to come from awake awareness in their work and how to foster this awareness in their clients. There is no book for therapists on this topic that illuminates in such depth and detail exactly how to conduct therapy from this paradigm."

Susan Campbell, PhD, author of *Getting Real* and
From Triggered to Tranquil

The Awakened Therapist

The Awakened Therapist is an accessible introduction to gestalt therapy through the lens of transpersonal counseling, one that offers a clear and profound account of how to bridge the gap between traditional counseling and spiritual transformation. Bringing new depths to the art of therapy, Harmony Kwiker provides a map for therapists to dismantle the old paradigm of therapist-as-expert and honor their clients' innate wisdom. The chapters seamlessly weave together elusive concepts of levels of awareness, subtle energy, and spiritual alignment with psychological concepts that are embedded in the theory and application of gestalt therapy. After reading this book, therapists will be inspired and energized while having more substantial breakthroughs with their clients.

Harmony Kwiker, MA, LPC, is a visiting instructor at Naropa University serving as lead gestalt faculty. She is the founder of the Institute for Spiritual Alignment, where she teaches the art of transpersonal counseling.

The Awakened Therapist

Spirituality, Consciousness, and Subtle Energy in Gestalt Therapy

Harmony Kwiker

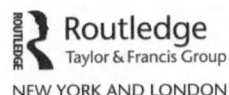

Routledge
Taylor & Francis Group

NEW YORK AND LONDON

Designed cover image: Getty Images

First published 2025
by Routledge
605 Third Avenue, New York, NY 10158

and by Routledge
4 Park Square, Milton Park, Abingdon, Oxon, OX14 4RN

Routledge is an imprint of the Taylor & Francis Group, an informa business

© 2025 Harmony Kwiker

The right of Harmony Kwiker to be identified as author of this work has been asserted in accordance with sections 77 and 78 of the Copyright, Designs and Patents Act 1988.

ISBN: 9781032862385 (hbk)
ISBN: 9781032862378 (pbk)
ISBN: 9781003521969 (ebk)

DOI: 10.4324/9781003521969

Typeset in Palatino, Futura, and Rockwell
by Deanta Global Publishing Services, Chennai, India

Access the Support Materials: www.routledge.com/9781032862378

Dedication

This book is dedicated to my father, Michael Kwiker, DO. Your unwavering faith in humanity's ability to awaken and heal inspires me over and over again. Thank you for paving the way for me to pave my own way.

▇ Contents

Figures

◼ Acknowledgments

I'd like to acknowledge the numerous wise healers who have been a clear mirror for me over the years. The profoundly transpersonal experiences I had in your presence have helped me to serve my clients and students with more clarity. Specifically, I'd like to thank Susan Nemcek, Jessika Siorai, Rachel Prairie, Aaron Overstreet, Lara Barber, Melissa Grace, Carolyn Eberle, and Colleen Buckman. I'd like to offer a deep bow to my mother, Elizabeth Kwiker (1950–2007), who was a powerful healer and wise seer. I'd also like to extend a heartfelt acknowledgment to my father, Michael Kwiker, DO, who has become one of my dearest allies. To my Spirit Mother, Bonnie Rascon, I'd like to thank you for your continued love and unending support; you are truly a sacred gift. To my husband, Christopher Arnold, thank you for your warm heart, clear mind, and persistent goodness. To my children, Mylah and Tobin, you are my greatest teachers and biggest motivation.

I would like to acknowledge Clarissa Cigrand, PhD, for holding our department at Naropa University with such care. Thank you to my editors, Meagan Estrella, MA, and Kim Minoso Smith, MA, who both brought so much wisdom and attention to detail into this offering. A special thank you to Nichole Xenos, PhD, for your wisdom and integrity as a social justice advocate and gestalt therapist. To my students, thank you for making me a better therapist and teacher through your curiosity and witness. And lastly, to my clients, I am forever honored to walk by your side as you do this deep and profound work.

About the Author

Harmony Kwiker, MA, LPC, is a psychotherapist and visiting instructor at Naropa University, where she serves as lead gestalt faculty. She is also the founder of the Institute for Spiritual Alignment, offering ongoing learning opportunities for therapists who are committed to awakening. In her first book, *Reveal: Embody the True Self Beyond Trauma and Conditioning*, Harmony vulnerably shares her story of transformation while simultaneously empowering readers to discover their truest selves. Her second book, *Align: Living and Loving from the True Self*, is a self-help book that offers a clear map of how to live from your true nature.

Preface

As therapists, we dedicate ourselves to the ongoing study of humanity's suffering and healing. We commit to understanding our own human condition, which allows us to bring our purest awareness into every moment with our clients. We do this not for our own ego fulfillment, nor do we do it simply for our client's benefit. We do this because we know that we are all connected, that none of us are liberated until all of us are liberated.

When I decided to study clinical psychology, I knew that my purpose and my career were one and the same. I was in touch with a deep inner knowing that I am a healer, that this is my purpose. I also knew that most people seek healing in traditional clinical settings, like counseling and psychotherapy. However, I had never experienced healing in a counseling or psychotherapy session. I wanted to. I sought it out and participated in it to the best of my ability. But every time I had a session, I left feeling more identified with my symptoms, and I had no positive shift in emotional, psychological, or spiritual transformation.

I recall a time in my life when I was overcome by the grief of losing my mother to cancer. I went to three different therapists trying to find someone who could help me process my grief. On my final attempt, I told the therapist that I was becoming so anxious that I couldn't leave my dog at home for more than an hour. Her reply was, "You know you can't do that forever." I was so heartbroken by this response. I was looking for a wise healer who could support me in honoring my grief as sacred. Instead of feeling held in my experience of grieving my mother, I felt shame for the strategy I created to help me soothe.

All too often in psychotherapy, the therapist holds space from the seat of the expert, guided by their personality and conditioned self. When the power differential is such that the therapist is the expert and the client needs to be fixed, a client's own innate wisdom and capacity to heal are often overridden by frameworks and ideals of "normal." Clinicians tend to interpret clients and attempt to rearrange ideas, which supersedes following a client's inherent intelligence as they find their way back to their innate wholeness.

So, while being a healer was my clear purpose, choosing psychotherapy as my career was not a clear choice. I knew the therapeutic relationship was a sacred one, but my experience as a client taught me how a counselor who lacks awareness of their own state of consciousness can harm a client and cause them to feel worse. Psychotherapists want to serve their clients to the best of their ability, and they hold a high bar for themselves. However, this high bar often prevents them from meeting their clients from their most awake, resourced Self.

As I entered graduate school, I wanted to explore a new way to transform psychotherapy. I knew that the therapeutic relationship mattered more than my interventions; however, I was not explicitly taught how to cultivate a healthy and dynamic therapeutic relationship. I was taught about the psychopathology of a client and how to evaluate their mental health. I was also taught ethical standards and communication skills. However, not one teacher mentioned my own state of consciousness as being important. Aside from a brief note on countertransference and transference, no one indicated that the place within myself that I guide therapy from mattered. I graduated without knowing the role of my own presence, alignment, and awareness in the therapy room.

As with any relationship, the therapeutic one can be either dynamic or dull, empowering or oppressive. Psychotherapy has the potential to facilitate the deepest repair in clients, and aside from the client's own inner and outer resources (such as resilience and social support), the therapist's presence influences the potency of what is possible within a session (Gelso and Carter, 1985; Norcross and Lambert, 2018).

The tenets of this book are that all people are whole, all symptoms are adaptive, and each person carries the wisdom within themselves that will guide their healing and transformation. Being a vessel for other people's healing and transformation requires that we stay in contact with the Source of healing as we hold space. We do this not because we believe we are *the* source of healing, but because being anchored within our own energy allows us to trust our client's inner wisdom. When a client is suffering, they don't need advice or sympathy—they need to find their way back home to their true nature. From an awakened state, we can be the reminder they need on their journey back to their True Self.

This book offers a bridge between traditional psychotherapy and transpersonal spiritual healing. Concepts from gestalt therapy are interwoven with transpersonal counseling, offering insight into the practice of guiding deep transformation. Awake awareness, unfinished business, polarities, transpersonal parts work, subtle energy, and more are explored in depth to support you in holding space for your clients from your most awake, resourced Self.

As the paradigm of psychotherapy moves from a colonized endeavor to a more spiritual exploration, therapists have the opportunity to support deep repair of collective suffering. In transpersonal counseling, spirituality is viewed as innate and integral to a person's health and healing (Miller, 2023). This is different from a person's religious beliefs or traditions, which are learned and acquired. Without imposing any of our own belief systems onto clients, we can honor our clients as sacred beings as they explore and reconnect to their wholeness and to their deepest truth.

To do this deep work as a clinician, we must also do this deep work as a person. We can only meet our clients as deeply as we meet ourselves. This does not mean that we need to be perfectly healed and know what to do in each moment. It simply means that if we are truly dedicated to our clients' healing and awakening, we are also dedicated to our own. As we heal into life together, our life becomes a prayer, where our existence contributes to restoring peace and balance to humanity.

Here are a few things to consider as you read this book:

♦ Concepts of spirituality are referred to as innate qualities, not religious ideology.
♦ Words that allude to this innate divinity are written with a capital letter to express reverence for this sacred quality. Words and phrases beginning with a capital include:
  ♦ Self or True Self, indicating the truest, most authentic place within a person.
  ♦ Source or Source That Beats Your Heart, indicating the sacred life-giving energy that precedes us.
♦ The subject "we" is used to reference the therapist. Occasionally, it is used for the collective experience of humanity. This is done deliberately to highlight the human condition.

- Gestalt therapy is the foundational theory from which spirituality, consciousness, and subtle energy are explored in the therapy room.
- Transpersonal counseling is embedded within gestalt therapy, and it is expanded upon as the place where intuitive and transcendent experiences support transformation.

Conscious Awareness and the Therapeutic Container

Chapter 1

Resting in Awareness

Therapists seek to offer their clients the most effective intervention, reflection, or modality to make the deepest healing possible. Although this effort is noble, it can also inhibit the quality of our presence. Striving to have the solutions to our clients' suffering is a manifestation of our persona. When we believe we are the rescuer of our clients' suffering, we deprive them of the opportunity to find their own way.

Dismantling the old paradigm of clinician-as-expert is essential in offering clients a truly sacred space to heal and find their way back to their true nature. When we position ourselves as the expert, we are more likely to be identified with our ordinary mind, which is our thought-based reality. From this identification, we are more prone to interpret and analyze our clients rather than meet them from our boundless true nature. Similarly, we are more likely to be unconscious to our own inner biases that reinforce our client's sense of disempowerment and fragmentation. Instead of trusting their inherent movement toward health, we manage their symptoms and engage with their thought-based reality.

Whichever modality we use, the lens through which we see our clients greatly affects what is possible in their therapeutic process. Our perception of our clients is a reflection of our own level of awareness, also known as our state of consciousness. When we embody higher levels of awareness, our presence reminds our clients of the place within themselves that is whole and infinite. Guided by the loving and boundless energy of our innate spirituality, our presence honors and invites this same quality within the client to come forth as the catalyst for their integration and healing.

Staying with our experience of the present moment, we can let go of any preconceived notions of what it means to be a therapist. Drawing from concepts of Zen Buddhism and Taoism, an awakened approach to counseling emphasizes the therapist's contemplative practices and state of consciousness as essential to our efficacy as a clinician (Gold & Zahm, 2018). Bringing a quality of presence that is both expansive and clear, we engage in the therapeutic relationship as a meditation on the here and now (Resnick, 1975). We open to our authentic expression in the therapy room and contact our clients from our whole self, which is called the dialogic relationship (Yontef, 1998). When fully participating in the therapeutic relationship, we affirm our clients' humanity as we navigate their inner world with them.

Without the illusions of our mind skewing our perceptions, our clients are provided with a relational matrix of compassionate and accurate witness to rediscover their true nature. Rather than interpreting a client's behavior, we invite our clients to experience themselves as they are, which is termed phenomenology (Merleau-Ponty & Smith, 2014). Phenomenology is

DOI: 10.4324/9781003521969-2

the exploration of the client's immediate experience, honoring this as the greatest authority in their process. The self-attunement of phenomenology facilitates self-responsibility, where clients discover how to stay present with themselves as they find their way through their distress and habitual patterns toward integration and regulation (Perls et al., 1951).

To let go of the mind and rest in awareness is a practice. Over time, we increase our capacity to open to the inherent intelligence within ourselves, the client, and the therapeutic container all at once. Influenced by our mindful presence and attention, clients increase their awareness and understanding by attuning to what is happening within themselves in the present moment. While this work is in service of the client's transformation, we also become more conscious and awake as we engage in the art of this profound therapy. In order to access the wisdom of this dynamic approach, we need to understand how transpersonal counseling and gestalt theory support this endeavor.

Beyond the Self

States of consciousness that are beyond the limits of personal identity are explored in *transpersonal* counseling (Friedman & Hartelius, 2015). Experiences beyond normal waking may be described as a mystical awareness, dream-like state, hypnotic state, or psychedelic experience (Cunningham, 2022). Transcendent transmissions in the form of images, words, and sensations may materialize spontaneously or with intentional practices. These expansive experiences are revered as healing and integrating of the inner divisions between the mental, emotional, physical, and spiritual aspects of a person's being (Walsh & Vaughan, 1993).

Transpersonal psychology and counseling view non-ordinary states of consciousness as normal and healthy (Cunningham, 2022). To hold a transpersonal therapeutic container, we must familiarize ourselves with the infinite wisdom of expanded consciousness. Time in nature, breathwork, yoga, meditation, and psychedelic-assisted therapy offer us the container to practice differentiating from our personality. In these experiences, we learn to rest in the vast awareness that is the bridge to the transpersonal.

Our normal waking state of consciousness is characterized by the ordinary mind, which includes our ego, personality, and conditioned self. At the level of the ordinary mind, everything is personal. From the way other people express themselves, to unmet needs and disappointments, our mind personalizes the world around us. Seeing people and the environment as separate causes us to experience life as a series of obstacles. Normal waking consciousness has us believe that we are our personality and that our thoughts are reality. Identification with our ordinary mind inhibits non-ordinary states from emerging. This is compounded by societal standards and expectations that normalize identification with the ordinary mind and pathologize non-ordinary states (Cunningham, 2022).

Although the ordinary mind is useful and important for navigating certain elements of life, it does not inspire the quality of presence and awareness that is needed to guide deep transformation. When we engage in the therapeutic process from our personality, we limit the healing potential of a session. In times of stress and dysregulation, the survival mechanism of our nervous system causes our access to higher consciousness to shut down (Miller, 2023). These are potent moments to practice mindfulness. Experiencing our dysregulation with loving compassion, we can shift from our thought-based reality to expanded states of consciousness.

The more we access transpersonal states in our own personal development, the more we increase our capacity to open to transcendent experiences in real time with our clients. We can delve into the transpersonal realm and engage in the therapeutic process from elevated states of consciousness. When our sense of identity extends beyond our individual self, we embrace the vast and infinite wisdom of life, humankind, psyche, and cosmos. This phenomenon is regarded as vital to our health and well-being, as well as to our contribution to the therapeutic process.

What Is Gestalt Therapy?

Gestalt therapy is a creative and experimental approach to counseling that emphasizes the sacred nature of the therapeutic relationship. As an intuitive and integrative approach to psychotherapy, it is influenced by a variety of traditions, including existential philosophy, Eastern religion, Reichian character analysis, Gestalt psychology, psychodrama, and psychoanalysis (Smith, 1976). Trusting that awareness is healing in and of itself, gestalt therapy weaves together these traditions and frameworks to create a dynamic therapeutic environment for clients to discover their way back home to their true nature.

The word *gestalt* loosely translates to *a unique patterning that forms a whole* (Smith, 1976). When elements of the human experience are mapped out into a single configuration, the whole of the formation is greater than the sum of its parts (Kaffka, 1935). The interplay between psychological phenomena, biological functions, spiritual wisdom, and environmental factors contribute to the forming of a gestalt. Together, they represent an integrated whole, with properties that are beyond the summation of the various elements.

When environmental factors cause a person's needs to go unmet, their experience is left incomplete, and a gestalt is not formed. The person then moves through the world struggling to resolve the unmet need. For example, a child who has a nightmare may go to their caregivers to seek comfort. If their caregivers are unwilling or unable to provide that comfort (which is an environmental factor), this experience of an unmet need could prevent a gestalt from forming. Since the experience is incomplete, the child may grow into an adult who does not ask for comfort or who attempts to get comfort in ways that cause them distress. The interdependency between a person and their environment holds the key to incomplete gestalten (Mann, 2021).

Gestalt therapy views the way a person adapts to these environmental factors as inherently wise. However, when the original circumstances are no longer present, continuing to engage in the adaptive strategies interrupts a person's ability to be fully present with themselves and others (Perls, 1973). The meditative quality of the therapeutic relationship elicits the client's adaptive strategies, which informs the therapeutic process and experimentation.

While largely a supportive presence to the client, gestalt therapists are also directive when we confront a client's patterns. This confrontation is in service of increasing awareness, coming into contact, and resolving unfinished business. In this context, a client can dissolve the illusions that are preventing them from seeing themselves as they really are. The clarity of this actuality, combined with their increased awareness, makes it possible for them to step into their autonomy and become self-responsible (Naranjo, 2004).

What Makes Gestalt Transpersonal?

Gestalt therapy is often taught under the umbrella of humanistic psychology, as it is a client-led approach to honoring human existence (Schneider et al., 2014). Humanistic psychology emphasizes a client's wholeness and increasing awareness as paramount to their self-actualization, which is aligned with gestalt principles. Concepts of authenticity, self-worth, and autonomy are also highlighted as clinically important to understanding a client's unique expression as a human being.

While gestalt therapy has elements of a humanistic approach embedded in its theory, it is more accurately described as a transpersonal methodology because we look beyond the client's personal identity (Naranjo, 2000). As clients process elements of their human experience, they begin to increase awareness of the inner constructs of their perceived identity. This makes it possible for them to integrate various aspects of themselves and embody their spiritual nature, experiencing themselves beyond their thought-based reality. When humanistic principles support a client in differentiating from their personality and opening to the mystical, transpersonal transformation can unfold.

Embedded in gestalt's creation is the Zen Buddhist concept of non-duality, which recognizes that beneath the diversity of human experience "there is a single, infinite and indivisible reality, whose nature is pure consciousness, from which all objects and selves derive their apparently independent existence" (Spira, 2022). Because the personality perceives the environment as separate from one's self, gestalt therapy utilizes awareness and creative experiments to offer clients a way to differentiate from their thought-based reality. This assists them in opening to the unifying consciousness that dwells within them, which is honored as the Source of their healing (Friedman & Hartelius, 2015).

As clients open to their innate spirituality, they are able to listen deeply to their intuitive senses as they are guided from within. We support them in exploring their inner mind-body process as they listen to the consciousness that resides within their sensations. We invite them to access and honor their intuitive senses, discovering their own deep truth as they return to their true nature. We also offer them space to access the mystical realm that rests beyond their personality, where they may hear the consciousness of their ancestors and access other dimensions.

Another transpersonal aspect of gestalt is the way the consciousness of the therapist contributes to the client's process. When facilitated by a therapist who meets the client beyond our personality and ego, deep exploration and healing unfold organically. Because we do not engage with the client's personality from our personality, we hold the container with a transpersonal, non-dual awareness where we do not see the client as a separate other.

Instead of interpreting or trying to figure out the client, we listen to their words, their expression, the subtle energy, as well as our experience of them in our own being. Our bodily sensations, impulses, and thoughts are viewed as resonant energy with what is occurring in the client. This is not the same as countertransference, where our personal feelings shape the way we interact with our clients. Coming into resonance is about being an energetic mirror, where our presence amplifies the places within the client that need to be integrated. When everything we experience in ourselves as we hold space for a client is honored as intuitive insight into their inner world, everything we experience within the session becomes part of the therapeutic process. This is only possible when we aren't personalizing our experience of the client or seeing them as a separate other.

When our wisdom and intuition interact with our client's wisdom and intuition, transpersonal transformation can unfold organically. Listening deeply to what is being communicated in the awareness field, we can hear our clients beyond the words they speak. Making room for each layer of consciousness to move through the client and through the container, the space for mystical experiences to transpire increases. This is, in part, what distinguishes transpersonal gestalt from other forms of talk therapy. The infinite possibilities inherent in this approach make it a dynamic and transcendent experience for both the therapist and the client.

Honoring the Sacred Boundary

From the ordinary mind, there is frequently an impulse to offer advice or tell a client what we believe is true. Similarly, there can be an impulse to lead a client to their healing or carry their pain for them. In these moments, we cross over the sacred boundary and miss the opportunity of meeting them in the I–Thou, where two whole beings engage authentically in relationship (Buber, 1958).

When therapists and clients actively and authentically engage each other in the here and now, a new relational dimension manifests (Buber, 1958). This sacred space where two (or more) whole individuals contact one another is known as an I–Thou relationship. In the I–Thou relationship, we open to awareness and recognize our clients as dynamic, living organisms. Seeing our clients as mysterious and sacred beings, we meet them in *the between*, where the relationship becomes greater than the individual offerings of those present. Philosopher Martin Buber (1958) described *the between* as a "bold leap into the experience of the other while simultaneously being transparent, present and accessible."

The I–Thou relationship is contrasted by the I–It relationship, where the other person is experienced as an object to be influenced or a means to get what we want (Buber, 1958). By not playing the role of the expert, offering advice, or trying to fix our clients, we are engaging with our clients as a divine *Thou*. Trusting that their inherent wisdom will guide their healing and transformation, we make room for their process to unfold in their own way and in their own time.

The sacred boundary exists within the I–Thou, where we do not impose our ideas and assumptions onto our clients. Instead, we honor our perception and stay curious about their deepest, most authentic truth and desire. We stay aligned within ourselves, and our presence invites the client to open to their alignment. We trust in their inherent wisdom as well as their process. When we try to do the work for them, we cross the sacred boundary and give our energy away, which leads to our depletion and burnout. Since this is their work to do, we hold space for them to find their way through their struggle.

Opening to Awareness

Instead of working to heal our clients' pain, we must expand our sense of identity beyond our individual self and open to the vast and infinite wisdom of awareness. Awareness is the expansive energy that has been with us always, even before our conception. It is beyond form and is already liberated and free (Gold & Zahm, 2018). It has the capacity to welcome all aspects of the human condition with love, and it is the bridge to integrating and transmuting even the most habitual, painful, and seemingly impermeable patterns.

The expansive nature of awareness allows us to encompass our experience, our client's experience, and the therapeutic relationship all at once. In addition, awareness allows us to access intuitive transmissions in the form of images, sensations, words, smells, and so on. Our mind supports this endeavor by tracking, remembering, and recalling various elements of the client's current and past experiences, mapping them into an organized whole.

Knowing that our mind does not hold the ultimate truth, we hold our perspective loosely. From this inner spaciousness, we offer our witness with the most clarity and neutrality possible. Acknowledging that what we see is from our perspective, our words are offered as a gift. While we share our reflections, we also stay curious to the client's perspective and experience. This synergy between therapist and client is a transpersonal experience, where our wisdom collaborates with our client's wisdom in service of their healing.

Tending to these micro elements of the present moment experience is made possible by opening into awareness. We cannot rely on the mind to track all of these elements at once, for it is limited by discrete bounds. Awareness, however, extends beyond the confines of the mind into the transpersonal realm of oneness with all of life.

When awareness guides the nuance of the therapeutic relationship, we experience an energizing meeting point between ourselves and our clients. From here, clarity and presence evoke the wisdom of self-responsibility. It is from this place that clients leave sessions feeling empowered and ready to meet life from their most authentic self. When the work-day is complete, the therapist leaves feeling like themselves, if not more awake and resourced for having met their clients in a way that is affirming of the wholeness of them both.

Signs of an Awakened Therapist

- ◆ Looks at their own conditioned patterns.
- ◆ Accesses the sensations in their body.
- ◆ Opens to intuitive transmissions.
- ◆ Respects the client's intuitive knowing.
- ◆ Sees the client as whole.
- ◆ Trusts the client's movement toward health.
- ◆ Holds no agenda for the client.
- ◆ Is aware of their own cultural lenses and biases.
- ◆ Holds no assumptions about what the client needs.
- ◆ Becomes aware when they want something for the client.
- ◆ Listens to the wisdom of the client's body.
- ◆ Stays fully present in the here and now.
- ◆ Sees the client as the expert of their own healing.
- ◆ Meets the client at the sacred boundary.
- ◆ Owns their perspective as theirs.
- ◆ Discovers what is true for their client.
- ◆ Feels more energized at the end of sessions because they are aligned.

Lessons from the Therapy Room

Like most psychotherapists, counselors, and coaches, I have a "helper" personality. My conditioned patterns are centered on prioritizing other people's needs, deferring to their opinions, and believing I'm responsible for their happiness. As a white, cisgender, heterosexual woman, my sense of self developed in a cultural context imbued by patriarchal ideologies and white privilege that I could not fully see or understand.

I was raised in Sacramento, CA, in a liberal household. My parents are old hippies who dedicated their lives to serving others. Although they were very loving, the unspoken expectations to be helpful, obliging, and fit standards of beauty set by the colonial patriarchy caused me to develop habits to fit into a box of conditioning that was both oppressive and inauthentic.

My propensity to accommodate others and betray myself was so deeply seated in shame and delusions of not being lovable that I hustled for approval from anyone and everyone— including my clients. As a new therapist, I wanted so badly to empower my clients and support their deepest healing. My eagerness, however, did not translate into effectiveness. In my newness, I wanted to prove my value, and I tried to carry their burdens for them. I thought I needed to have all the answers, and I felt deeply insecure that I, in fact, did not hold the solution to their pain. I thought they needed me to be an expert, and I was afraid of failing them.

My limitations were not for lack of training or effort, but because my conditioned patterns guided my interactions with others. Beyond my training as a psychotherapist, I was very committed to contemplative practices, including meditation. I had been practicing Transcendental Meditation since I was six, I had taught yoga for many years, and I had experienced various degrees of awakening at different stages in my life. Alone on my meditation cushion, I could access vast expansive awareness. However, when relating with other people, my identity was firmly seated in my individual sense of self, and I was guided by ordinary awareness.

When I finally realized that my eagerness to please and accommodate was preventing me from confronting the incongruences within my clients, I became motivated to find a new way. With this fresh insight, I had a revelation: My normal waking consciousness was not capable of guiding deep transformation. I realized that if I wanted to open to awareness in the presence of my clients, I needed my personality to stay outside of the therapy room.

I decided that before each session I would meditate for ten minutes to connect with my Self. Then, before entering my office, I would say to my personality, "You are not allowed in this session. You are not capable of guiding deep transformation. I'll be back for you when I'm done."

Uncomfortable at first, I felt naked without my personality. However, this was the exact discomfort I needed to feel in order to open to awareness. I learned how to co-create profound therapy sessions that were beyond what my ordinary mind could conceive. This was the beginning of my ability to guide a transpersonal counseling session. Every day since has been a continuation of learning, deepening, and co-creating with my clients.

Exercise: Shifting to Awake Awareness

The ability to recognize when we are asleep to our true nature supports our ability to shift from our ordinary to awake awareness. Awake awareness is different from attention. Attention is the ability to shift focus from one thing to another, such as from our thoughts to our sensations. When we place our attention on a particular sensation in our body or the narratives of our mind, this attention can support us in turning on the light of awareness.

There are three stages in the practice of shifting to awake awareness: 1) Notice your mind, 2) come into direct experience, and 3) open to the expansive consciousness of your energy.

Notice Your Mind

◆   To begin, close your eyes and notice the thoughts in your mind. Without trying to stop your thoughts or interpret them, simply notice that you are thinking.

- With your inner eye, bring attention to the quality of the energy in your mind. Is it dense? Is it scattered? Is it looping? Or something else?
- Focus on the energetic quality of your mind. Experience your mind and welcome it as it is.

Come into Direct Experience

- Direct your attention down into your belly. At first, you may be looking down from your mind into your belly, as if you were shining a flashlight into your abdomen.
- Practice letting go of your thoughts and come into the consciousness that exists in your belly. Without trying to figure out if you're doing it correctly, just let go and open to your awareness as it exists in your belly. Notice if the energy in your belly is empty or full, dense or light, big or small. Be the inherent wisdom that exists within your belly.

Open to the Expansive Consciousness of Your Energy

- From your belly, begin to expand outward. Sense into the infinite, formless energy of awareness. This is the consciousness that has been with you since before your conception and will be with you long after you leave this body. Take a few breaths and explore the liberated freedom of this awareness.
- When you open your eyes, bring this awareness with you. Practice this often, to anchor yourself into awareness itself.

References

Buber, M. (1958). *I and thou*. Charles Scribner and Sons.

Cunningham, P. (2022). *Introduction to transpersonal psychology: Bridging spirit and science*. Routledge.

Friedman, H., & Hartelius, G. (2015). *The Wiley-Blackwell handbook of transpersonal psychology* (1st ed.). Wiley-Blackwell.

Gold, E., & Zahm, S. (2018). *Buddhist psychology & gestalt therapy integrated: Psychotherapy for the 21st century*. Metta Press.

Kaffka, K. (1935). *Principles of gestalt psychology*. Harcourt, Brace.

Mann, D. (2021). *Gestalt therapy: 100 key points and techniques*. Routledge.

Merleau-Ponty, M., & Smith, C. (2014). *Phenomenology of perception*. Humanities Press.

Miller, L. (2023). *The awakened brain*. Random House Publishing Group.

Naranjo, C. (2004). *Gestalt therapy: The attitude and practice of an atheoretical experientialism*. Crown House Pub Ltd.

Perls, F. (1973). *The gestalt approach and eye witness to therapy* (1st ed.). Science and Behavior Books, Inc.

Perls, F., Hefferline, R., & Goodman, P. (1951) *Gestalt therapy: Excitement and growth in the human personality*. Souvenir Press.

Resnick, S. (1975). Gestalt therapy as a meditative practice. In J. Stevens (Ed.), *Gestalt Is* (pp. 223–228). Real People Press.

Schneider, K. J., Pierson, J. F., & Bungental, J. (2014). *The handbook of humanistic psychology: Theory, research, and practices*. Sage Publications.

Smith, E. (1976). The roots of gestalt therapy. In E. Smith (Ed.), The growing edge *of* gestalt *therapy* (pp. 3–35). Gestalt Journal Press.

Spira, R. (2022). *You are the happiness you seek: Uncovering the awareness of being*. Sahaja Press.

Walsh, R., & Vaughan, F. (1993). *Paths beyond ego: The transpersonal vision (New Consciousness Reader)*. TarcherPerigee.

Yontef, G. (1998). Dialogic gestalt therapy. In L. S. Greenberg, J. C. Watson, & G. Lietaer (Eds.), *Handbook of experiential psychotherapy* (pp. 82–102). The Guilford Press.

Chapter 2

Understanding Levels of Awareness

Therapists and clients arrive to sessions inhabiting varying levels of awareness. As therapists, our level of awareness affects our ability to stay present and engaged in the therapeutic relationship. It affects our emotional regulation, how we see our clients, where we direct attention, and what interventions we choose. This all has a direct impact on what is possible for a client in a session.

A client's level of awareness influences the way they relate to their environment and their *self*, which is characterized by their impulses, thoughts, behaviors, and personality (Skottun & Kruger, 2021). In lower levels of awareness, clients feel powerless to effect their own healing and transformation. Attempting to change from the same level of awareness that creates their distress, a client's progress is limited by their own state of consciousness.

Awareness rests on a continuum, from low to high. The more awareness we have of our inner and outer experiences, the more access we have to higher levels of consciousness. It may seem that our level of awareness is haphazard, as if it were outside of our own influence. However, with practice, both ourselves and our clients can learn to move into higher levels of awareness throughout the course of a therapeutic cycle.

The Alchemy of Awareness

Awareness is the most valuable resource in our clients' transformation. Being seen with clarity through our awareness, they can begin to understand the inner patterns of what they have been tolerating within themselves. When what is familiar to them is accurately seen through our witness, their awareness begins to shift, soften, and alchemize their inner patterns.

A client's sense of self is an organized process that is constantly changing as they interact with their environment (Perls, 1973). To awaken a client's innate movement toward health, direct contact with a therapist who embodies higher levels of awareness is vital. The therapist's state of consciousness interacts with a client's developing sense of self, reminding

DOI: 10.4324/9781003521969-3

them of the place within that holds the answers to their suffering. When their higher levels of awareness ignite their healing, they are guided by their own innate wisdom. From this place, the work they do in a session will be aligned and lasting.

Because we do not hold a goal of changing our clients, we encourage our clients to become more self-aware as they process in the here and now. As they struggle with their own perceived limitations, we contact them in each facet and expression as the layers of their inner world emerge. Our unwavering presence and compassion models the principles of nonviolence, where even the most antagonistic inner critic is honored as adaptive and seen with the clarity of awareness.

Throughout this experience, a client begins to increase their level of awareness. They move from identification with their *self* to curiosity about what their patterns are communicating. This increased curiosity facilitates our client's ability to move from judgment to compassion, resistance to openness, clinging to surrender, and distress to peace. Where they were once contracted around their inner experience, they move to an expanded state of awareness, which is both spacious and self-responsible. The synergy between the therapist's and the client's awareness evokes this alchemy, where the client's distress seems to magically transform into contentment.

Level 1: Ordinary Awareness

The normal waking state of consciousness is called *ordinary awareness*. Ordinary awareness is guided by our thought-based reality, which is comprised of our impulses, thoughts, behaviors, and personality. This is the lowest level of awareness, and it takes the least amount of effort or intention to maintain. Believing that truth and reality exist in the mind, ordinary awareness has us put forth tremendous mental effort searching for a narrative that will hopefully offer a solution.

As clients interpret themselves, their body sensations, and other people through the mind, they perpetuate their own distress. Ideas *about* themselves or what they *should* be experiencing keep them out of presence as they languish in ordinary awareness. *Aboutism* is a gestalt term that refers to the propensity to talk *about* something, retreating into the mind rather than fully experiencing themselves (Perls, 1973). A person who is highly influenced by the world of science is more likely to maintain an ordinary awareness characterized by *aboutism*. *Shouldism*, on the other hand, is a term designated for the way a person creates a fantasy of how they think they *should* be. A person who is highly influenced (either consciously or unconsciously) by religion is more prone to an ordinary awareness influenced by *shouldism*.

Aboutisms and *shouldisms* are a sort of mental trap set by the mind that expresses a person's unresolved experiences. When unresolved experiences are left unexamined and unprocessed, inner conflicts and anguish keep a client feeling stuck. It is not our intention to vilify or vanquish the ordinary mind. Ordinary awareness is extremely valuable in navigating the world, as it retrieves memories and supports daily functioning. We simply want to support clients in differentiating from their ordinary awareness to see their thoughts more clearly.

To support clients in differentiating from their thought-based reality, we must first understand the way this level of awareness shows up in a session. *When a client is in a state of distress and feels trapped in that distress, they are experiencing an ordinary state of awareness.* Some of the ways ordinary awareness is expressed in a session include:

- ♦ **Id:** A person's id consists of their unconscious impulses, urges, and desires. Emotional impulses and sexual desire can seem to be beyond the client's logic and reason. Although below the level of conscious thinking, these primitive instincts influence the content of the client's ordinary awareness.

- ♦ **Personality:** Clients who are identified with their personality have thoughts that limit their expression and choice. Oftentimes, the personality holds habitual patterns that cause them to give their power away, resent others, feel responsible for others, and so on. Attachment wounds are almost always expressed through a personality.

- ♦ **Ego:** A person's ego is their sense of self-esteem and self-importance. When a person is identified with their ego, they typically hold pride-based identifications that are an attempt to give them a sense of value (Heller & LaPierre, 2012). This is the part of the mind that wants to control. When they are identified with their ego, there are shadow-identifications that a person resists within themselves, such as misused power or disowned desire.

- ♦ **Attachment Wounds:** Attachment wounds are emotional wounds created in relationship with their primary caregiver during the development of their personality. When the client believes the narratives that they have created based on past relational harm, they feel distress when their narratives about themselves and others are present.

- ♦ **Narrative Creation:** When a client is identified with their thought-based reality, they will frequently talk *about* themselves or how they think they *should* be when making sense of the world. They hold onto these stories, trying to anchor themselves into existence, struggling to come into presence and let go of their conceptualizations.

- ♦ **The Body:** Physical sensations and direct experiences with the body are typically rejected by someone who is hyper-identified with their ordinary mind. The body is seen as an object and often becomes desensitized as they loop in thought. Even when they do turn toward the body, they still try to interpret or analyze their felt experience.

- ♦ **Internalized Societal Factors:** In ways that are both apparent and obscure, societal factors influence a client's ordinary awareness. Gender norms of the dominant culture, systemic oppression, world events, political rhetoric, and other environmental influences inform the way a client makes sense of themselves and the world. Unknowingly, this may be a large contribution to the client's distress.

Level 2: Subtle Awareness

Direct experience of the here and now is the bridge from ordinary awareness into *subtle awareness.* Subtle awareness is the ability to sense, perceive, and experience the inner and outer dimensions of the human experience, also known as interoception (Porges, 2017). When a client ignores their body and orients toward their thoughts, the wisdom of their subtle awareness goes unnoticed. Through the acceptance of their present moment experience, they begin to sensitize to their subtle awareness, which dwells right beneath their normal waking state.

When a therapist pays more attention to the client's expression than to the stories they share, we are tracking the client's ordinary and subtle awareness at the same time (Kurtz, 1990). When invited to attune to the subtle, a client's bodily sensations give the ordinary mind a place to anchor in the present moment. From this presence, clients are able to shift from thought-based reality to awareness-based reality, where their subliminal mind opens to insight, images, epiphanies, and previously forgotten memories (Milton, 1980).

Clients may also resist turning toward their direct experience as they continue to orient toward their thought-based reality. It is common for a client to try to interpret the subtle in an attempt to cling to their mind. Even the client's impulses to interpret, cling, and resist have subtle experience imbued within them that we can attune to as their therapist. Contacting them where they are with our subtle awareness brings a gentle quality of presence that supports the client in increasing awareness of the way they relate to themselves. These moments create openings for the client to become more present with themselves as they are.

This mindful approach to the therapeutic relationship is called the *awareness continuum,* where we use present moment, open questions to support self-awareness of what is happening in the here and now (Naranjo, 2004). The following questions are examples of the awareness continuum: "What are you noticing right now?" "What do you notice in your body?" "What do you notice about your breath?" (This practice is explored in the exercise at the end of this chapter.)

There is an art to using the awareness continuum in sessions, which is influenced by the therapist's *why* for utilizing this intervention. Some reasons to use the awareness continuum include: Increasing self-awareness, coming into direct experience, interrupting the ways in which a client disrupts contact with the present moment, nervous system regulation, honoring the client's organismic self-regulation, and gathering information about the client.

How a client responds to the awareness continuum offers us tremendous insight into their state of consciousness. If they seem unsettled or confused by the invitation, we have the opportunity to gain deeper understanding about how they relate to their present moment experience. We can meet them in the confusion from our own subtle awareness, and this discomfort becomes the entry point into therapeutic transformation.

When a client has experienced prolonged complex trauma, they may be desensitized to their somatic sensations. The feeling of nothing in the body is important to contact from subtle awareness. Where the ordinary mind may be distressed by this disconnection from the body, we view it as a wise mechanism of the nervous system. When honored with subtle awareness, disconnection becomes the entry point to reconnecting to one's Self. When we ask a client what they notice in their body, if they say "nothing," it is important we don't assume what "nothing" means. Turning toward nothing, we can ask the client if they feel numb or fuzzy or hollow or something else. By coming into direct experience with "nothing," the client begins to sensitize to their inner experience. Similarly, if the mind is their access point, we can invite them to attune to their mind with subtle awareness.

When a client contacts and experiences their distress in the here and now, they enter into subtle awareness, where they begin to gain wisdom from the distress itself. From subtle awareness, a few things occur:

- ♦ They begin to learn how to regulate their nervous system. The body houses the nervous system, and our thinking brain is not connected to our nervous system regulation.
- ♦ When a client opens up to the sensations in their body, they learn how to be available for themselves. They become more in touch with their actual lived experience rather than their narratives. This, in turn, supports them in becoming more self-responsible.
- ♦ They learn to become a secure base for themselves, repairing their attachment system in deep and lasting ways.
- ♦ They become present with themselves. All healing happens in the present moment. This access to the here and now is essential for their transformation.
- ♦ They may have spontaneous thoughts from the subliminal mind that offer insight into their patterns of distress.

Level 3: Awake Awareness

From the present moment state of subtle awareness, we begin to awaken to the inherent wisdom of organismic self-regulation, where we consciously respond to our needs (Korb et al., 2002). This self-regulation makes it possible to enter into the liberated and infinite energy of our deepest dimension, known as *awake awareness*. Awake awareness is the loving presence of the fundamental core of one's being that supports an integrated sense of self (Kelly, 2015).

When a client is ready to enter into this level of awareness, they let go of their thought-based reality and open to awareness-based knowing, where their inherent wisdom dwells. From their connection to this profound inner resource, they begin to navigate their inner matrix with an understanding of what they need from themselves to integrate and heal, allowing every part of themselves to be touched by this loving and welcoming quality. Paradoxically, in loving what previously caused them distress, they organically transmute what they formerly struggled with. This is known as the *paradoxical theory of change*, where change occurs when a client stops trying to be something they are not and fully embodies who they are (Perls, 1973).

As the dialogic relationship requires that both the therapist and the client express their experiences and observations as two whole beings, the therapist's state of consciousness

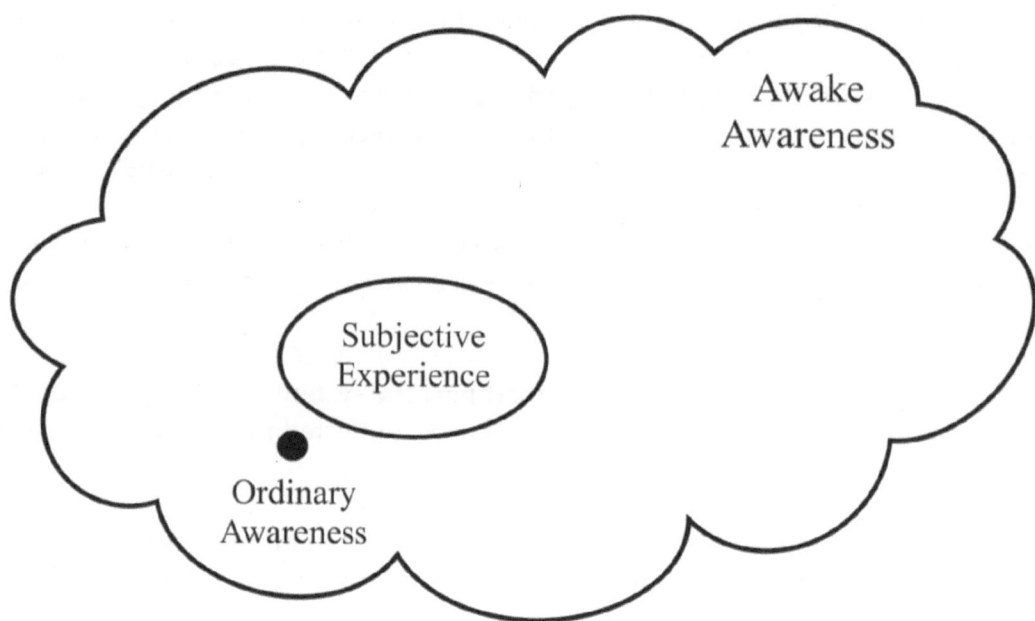

Figure 2.1 Awake Awareness

influences the client's ability to access awake awareness. If we are practiced in moving into an awake aware state throughout the course of a session, clients can awaken from even the most chronic and persistent patterns. Although we may begin a session from our ordinary mind, intentionally coming into direct experience and opening to awareness enables a transpersonal therapeutic relationship.

When we accurately reflect the client's present moment experience back to them from our expanded state of consciousness, they begin to see their habitual thoughts and patterns through the light of awareness. Through a combination of our presence in the dialogic relationship, our state of consciousness, and our present moment interventions, we affirm the client's wholeness. By trusting that they have the inner resourcing of awake awareness within them already, we honor that they hold the solutions to their own struggles.

Awareness is what allows our clients to understand their automatic habits as well as their environment, making it possible for them to engage with life from a more authentic place within themselves. Instead of reacting to their environment or habitually using adaptive survival strategies, a client is empowered with choice and self-responsibility.

In Figure 2.1, we can see that from the perspective of the ordinary awareness, our present moment experience (which may include fear, anger, pain, excitement, and so on) seems quite large, maybe even insurmountable. From awake awareness, however, whatever is present in this moment can be welcomed with loving and compassion. Figure 2.1

When a client is able to genuinely accept their distress with love and self-compassion, they transmute their distress into healing with awake awareness. Some ways to support a client to occupy the boundless energy of their awake awareness are as follows:

♦   Ask them awareness continuum questions that are inspired by our own attuned awareness, bringing attention to aspects of their inner world that may be energetically blocked or ignored.

- Ask them, "If this sensation had a voice, what would it say?" This allows the client to open to the wisdom of their body and experience a flow state with their own energy.
- Ask them, "What does this sensation need from you right now?" This gives them the opportunity to increase their awareness and be loving with themselves.
- Invite them to see their pain and continue to shine the light of awareness onto this experience. "Without trying to fix it, change it, or figure it out, just notice it as a loving witness." In being witnessed, the sensation begins to shift.
- Invite them to wrap the sensation or thought with validation and love.
- Invite them to close their eyes and turn toward themselves. When the eyes are closed, awareness of the inner experience is increased.
- Invite them to follow their breath, using the breath as a bridge from contraction to expansion.

Level 4: True Self Awareness

As we open to awake awareness, we have the ability to navigate our inner world with self-compassion and innate wisdom. Feeling more like ourselves than we do when we are hyper-identified with our ordinary awareness, we reconnect with our true nature. Connected to the purity of our essence, we may naturally enter into *True Self awareness*, which is the transpersonal experience of being one with everything.

True Self awareness is the consciousness that dwells within all of life, where there is no separation, no good or bad, and no need to control. It is the spiritual essence of a person's wholeness, a way of "being and experiencing what comes about through awareness of a transcendent dimension" (Elkins, 2015). Being one with all of life does not mean that we do not have differences, such as racial identities, personal histories, and so on. However, from this state of consciousness, we touch the place of oneness, where the egoic delusions of the individual identity dissolve, and our waking state becomes illuminated by the mystical and the transcendent.

When a client opens to True Self awareness, they integrate all aspects of themselves, where they enter into their spiritual nature, shadow, personality, compassionate heart, and more all at once. They also feel kindness toward themselves and others, and have a clarity where they were previously clouded with narratives. They accept their past and see the wisdom for how they survived and adapted. They feel compassion for the people in their lives without objectifying them as something to fulfill their own dissatisfaction. Interconnectedness becomes their state of being.

A client cannot be guided to True Self awareness, for this is a natural and spontaneous expression of their health. Organically, a client finds their way to their True Self in their own way and at their own time. *When a client organically enters into oneness, they integrate all aspects of themselves and embody their spiritual nature with True Self awareness.*

Some indicators that a client embodies their True Self include the following:

♦ They feel a sense of peace.
♦ Their mind is quiet and their body is regulated.
♦ They feel a sense of acceptance for their life's journey.
♦ They feel a sense of compassion toward their acquired ideas about themselves and the world.
♦ They are connected to their true Source of love within themselves and stop looking to others to affirm their worth or value.
♦ They feel open to the unknown of their journey ahead.
♦ They embody *self-responsibility*, where they have the *ability* to *respond* to their inner and outer experiences from their True *Self*.

Becoming a Clear Mirror

The deepest repair of the client's healing can begin to actualize when they are accurately mirrored in the eyes of the therapist. With our whole being, we communicate to our clients that we hear, see, feel, and sense the entirety of their experience, even beyond the words they've said. Attunement is the process by which we bring all aspects of our client's experience into harmony with one another (Merriam-Webster, 2024). The clarity of our attunement allows us to meet our clients where they are while also illuminating their shadow and blind spots. As a compassionate witness, we see their distress, their shadow, and their wholeness.

To be a clear mirror, we must observe and witness our clients as they are. Without our own agenda, projections, or interpretations, we cultivate the capacity to expand our awareness. To see our clients through the lens of awareness, it is helpful to have a baseline of how we feel in our bodies before we step into a session. When we are connected to our own sense of self, it becomes easier to recognize when our experience during a session—including thoughts, sensations, intuitions, and so on—belongs to us or our client. Embodying our individual experience is paradoxically necessary to understanding our experience *of* our client.

Being fully present in the here and now and engaged in therapy from full contact with ourselves produces a therapeutic space where everything we experience within the container belongs to the client. Even a seemingly extraneous or fleeting thought or emotion that we experience becomes an invaluable element of the client's full gestalt. For example, if we are sitting with a client and suddenly feel fear in our system, our mind may try to figure out why fear is present. The narrative we create may be about ourselves or our client. We may question, "Did I say the right thing?" or "Why is the client turning away from fear?"

Without personalizing our expereince, we can simply make room for the energetic quality of fear to be welcomed into the therapeutic space. We may offer, "I'm not sure why, but my attention just went to fear. What do you notice when I say that?" By naming fear explicitly, we welcome the quality of fear without denying it or making meaning of it. Perhaps the client is aware of fear in the moment or perhaps they are not. Either way, we are not holding the fear of the session in our bodies, *and* we are using what is present in our awareness therapeutically.

When we ignore our own inner observations of our felt sense as we sit with a client, we decrease our ability to be a clear mirror. By not voicing our implicit experience of our clients, we end up processing their emotions for them, which is not only ineffective but also leads to burnout. Similarly, when we perceive a pattern of thinking, feeling, behaving, or energetically moving in our client and do not name it, we decrease our client's ability to see themselves clearly. Because they are accustomed to their experience of themselves, they can become desensitized or oblivious to their own way of being.

Our experience of what is happening *right now* in the therapeutic relationship offers more insight than narratives our clients share. How we feel as we sit with a client can inform our understanding of how they feel and/or how the people in their life feel in relationship to them. Finding language that is contactful and honors our experience of our client increases our effectiveness and the clarity of the container we create. By our explicitly naming what we observe, their implicit ways of being are brought into the awareness field, which increases our clients' ability to process what is theirs to process.

If we see or sense a pattern in the client and try to analyze them or fix them, we are unconsciously communicating that we are the expert and undermine their access to their own healing. In these moments, the client's amygdala senses judgment, and we become a threat to their nervous system (Dion, 2018). Similarly, if we see a pattern in our client and do not reflect it, our presence is incongruent. In these moments, we again become a threat to their nervous system. (We will explore more on threats to the amygdala in later chapters.)

If we do not make the implicit explicit, we are more likely to try to change the client by offering advice or leading them to the solution to their distress. Our mirroring offers the client's words and expressions back to them imbued with the light of awareness. Aside from supporting the client's clarity, this keeps the container clean and reinforces that this is the client's work to do. Each time we offer a client their words back to them through the filter of awake awareness, they can deepen into their own healing process. This reinforces the sacred boundary, where our presence honors their autonomy.

Lessons from the Therapy Room

As a new psychotherapist, I worked hard for my clients. I saw the beauty of their wholeness, and I wanted them to see that in themselves, too. With the best of intention, I tried to lead my clients to their healing. Instead of meeting them where they were, I left the present moment and unknowingly projected a *shouldism* onto my clients, attempting to guide them to how I thought they should be.

Fortunately, I was attuned enough to realize that my presence caused more therapeutic rupture than contact. I was beginning to recognize that if I were to truly honor the pillar of nonviolence, I needed to fully welcome clients as they were. This was around the time when I started leaving my personality outside of the therapy room. During this exercise, I started to recall memories from childhood, specifically moments when I spontaneously saw the subtle energy of my mom's breathwork clients.

Both of my parents were holistic healers, and as a child, I was exposed to many different transpersonal forms of healing. My mom worked from home, so her breathwork and coaching practice was a normal part of my daily life. As a six-year-old child, I would see that before a session, her clients seemed heavy with a dark, murky vapor. After their breathwork sessions, their energy seemed light and fluffy and supple.

Because nobody was talking about subtle energy, I tried to figure out what I was seeing on my own. Before a session with my mom, I would ask her clients to lie down on the couch. I would put a crystal on the part of their body that seemed to be holding blocked energy, and I instructed them to breathe deeply.

Somehow, this gift lay dormant for years, and then one day as I was sitting with a client it came back to me. I was listening to my client talk about how her primary caregiver in childhood couldn't see her for who she was. Her posture was slumped over, and she seemed heavy with grief. I listened with empathy, and then I asked her what she was aware of in her body. "I'm so sad," she said as she cried.

I could see that she was sad, and I had my attention on her heart center, which had the energetic appearance of condensed dark gray emotional energy. "What do you notice in your heart?" I asked.

She closed her eyes and looked within. "My heart feels so heavy, like there's a hard almond in the center of my chest," she said.

The confirmation of the condensed energy in her heart center was enough insight for me to begin to trust my metaphysical eyes. Without projecting my intuition onto my client, I collaboratively used my perception to increase awareness in the therapeutic container.

"I'd like to invite you to keep your awareness on the almond shape in your heart. Without trying to change it or figure it out, just let it know that you see it, that you see what it's holding," I suggested.

As tears streamed down her face, her heart seemed to slowly soften, and her body seemed to unfold and lighten.

"I'm wondering if there is anything your heart needs from you right now?" I asked.

"Just this," she responded. "Just more love and attention."

"Take all the time you need," I invited. "Give your heart all the love and attention you need."

Her breath began to deepen, and she sighed with relief. As her energy began to move, I realized that her inner knowing had a wisdom that supported her own self-regulation. She was able to move through her experience with grace, not because I employed some technique, but because we both opened up to subtle awareness. This present moment, direct experience opened the door for her to access her awake awareness, where she had the capacity to be loving with the pain she was holding.

Exercise: Awareness Continuum

The *awareness continuum* is a tool to support the client's natural unfolding of awareness, presence, and contact (Naranjo, 2004). Clients discover their own patterns by themselves, for themselves, through the awareness continuum (Perls, 1973). This self-discovery is considered necessary for true change to manifest.

Aside from increasing the client's awareness, the awareness continuum offers insight for the therapist that makes it possible to follow the energy of the client. As we learn about the inner world of the client, we can pace the session, co-regulate, and keep the client within the window of tolerance, where there is some arousal and they can digest and integrate their emotions (Seigel, 2020).

The present moment is our home-base in a session, and the awareness continuum is one tool that invites a client back into presence. It is not a quick or rote filler question. It is a very intentional invitation to the client to awaken to their own experience. As the client shares their stories and narratives, the therapist pays more attention to the client than to their stories. While the stories are important and are utilized in the mapping of the client's inner world (which we will discuss in a later chapter), the inner mind–body connection of the here and now is invited into the session with the awareness continuum.

Awareness Continuum

What are you noticing right now?
What are you aware of right now?
What do you notice as you say that?
What do you notice in your body?
What do you notice on the level of sensation?
What's pulling the attention of your mind right now?
What do you notice about yourself right now?
What do you notice in (this specific body part)?
What do you notice about your breath?
What do you notice when I say that?

Find a practice partner, set the timer for six minutes, and only use the awareness continuum. With your attuned eye, ask present moment, open questions that invite your practice client into presence and deeper contact with themselves.

For example:

THERAPIST: "What are you noticing in your body right now?"
CLIENT: "I just keep thinking about work."
THERAPIST: "What do you notice on the level of sensation when you say that?"
CLIENT: "I don't feel sensation, except for my shoulders are tight."
THERAPIST: "Tell me more about your shoulders."

References

Dion, L. (2018). *Aggression in play therapy: A neurobiological approach for integrating intensity.* W. W. Norton & Company.

Elkins, D. (2015). *The human elements of psychotherapy: A nonmedical model of emotional healing* (1st ed.). American Psychological Association.

Heller, L., & LaPierre, A. (2012). *Healing developmental trauma: How early trauma affects self-regulation, self-image, and the capacity for relationships.* North Atlantic Books.

Kelly, L. (2015). *Shift into Freedom.* Sounds True.

Korb, M. P., Gorrell, J., & Van De Riet, V. (2002). *Gestalt therapy: Practice and theory* (2nd ed.). The Gestalt Journal Press.

Kurtz, R. (1990). *Body-centered psychotherapy: The hakomi method.* LifeRhythm.

Milton, H. (1980). *The collected papers of Milton H. Erickson on hypnosis, complete 4 volume set (nature of hypnosis and suggestion; hypnotic alteration of sensory, perceptual and psychophysiological processes; hypnotic investigation; innovative hypnotherapy)* (American 1st ed.). Irvington Publishers.

Naranjo, C. (2004). *Gestalt therapy: The attitude and practice of an atheoretical experientialism.* Crown House Pub Ltd.

Perls, F. (1973). *The Gestalt approach and eye witness to therapy* (1st ed.). Science and Behavior Books, Inc.

Porges, S. W. (2017). *The pocket guide to the polyvagal theory: The Transformative power of feeling safe.* W.W. Norton & Company.

Seigel, D. (2020). *Aware: The Science and Practice of Presence - The Groundbreaking Meditation Practice.* TarcherPerigee.

Skottun, G., & Kruger, A. (2021). *The theory of self in Gestalt therapy.* Routledge.

Chapter 3

Awareness of Cultural Lenses

Bringing higher levels of awareness to the therapy room includes being conscious of the cultural and racial identities that are present, which include our own, our clients', and those embedded in the modalities we use. Because the field of psychotherapy was created through a Eurocentric lens, we must acknowledge the way psychology and psychotherapy contribute to the ongoing wounds of colonialism. From systems of diagnosis to evidence-based practices, the field of psychotherapy has failed to tell a "complete and accurate story of why we are sick and how we get well" (Mullan, 2023).

Gestalt therapy was created in the late 1930s by Fritz Perls, Laura Perls, and Paul Goodman. As a groundbreaking approach to psychotherapy, gestalt revolutionized how clinicians engage in the therapy process. Holism, spirituality, psychodrama, phenomenology, mindful awareness, field theory, and authentic engagement in the I–Thou all contributed to the first therapy theory to honor the client's innate wisdom and natural movement toward health. By prioritizing process over pathology, in many ways the foundation for a decolonized approach to counseling was being created in the inception of gestalt therapy.

Although the advancement of psychotherapy was catapulted with gestalt, awareness of the way colonialism and patriarchy influenced the theorists, and thus the theory, appears to be unaccounted for in the early writing about gestalt (Perls et al., 1951; Perls, 1978, 1992). The language used in those early text books illuminated the societal norms of the time, including the use of he/him pronouns as the all-purpose pronouns and assumptions about gender roles. Since internalized white supremacy and internalized misogyny were not addressed by the theorists, the unconscious biases of the culture and era they lived within can be presumed to be embedded in gestalt.

Each one of us carries our own internalized ideas from the environment we exist within. Unless we examine the views we have adopted from society, we bring these unconscious ideas with us into our work as a therapist. A gestalt session is only as anti-racist as the therapist who is leading the session. In its purest form, the pillars of gestalt are culturally sensitive and compatible with a variety of cultural identities. However, the expression of these pillars is dependent on how they are held and expressed by the clinician.

Colonialism has been the source of harm at such a large scale, and it is the therapist's ethical duty to recognize the effect of colonialism within themselves, their clients, and the approach they use. It is not enough to simply do no harm; we must lovingly shine the light of awareness on the wound of colonialism so we can better understand the roots of symptoms and suffering for all people. If we do not talk about the harm caused by separation from land,

DOI: 10.4324/9781003521969-4

resources, ancestry, and a sense of belonging, we perpetuate the root of suffering imposed by racialized systems of oppression (Mullan, 2023). In order for psychotherapy to be a place for all people to experience true healing and liberation, we need to "look beyond attachment wounds and examine the wound of colonialism" (Mullan, 2023).

Microaggressions and Internalized Racism

Awareness of cultural lenses requires mindful attention to *internalized racism*, which is the "internalization of the racist stereotypes, values, images and ideologies perpetuated by the white dominant society about one's racial group" (Pyke, 2010). Ideas of superiority and inferiority are constructs that cause a disconnection from one's own sense of humanity, causing psychological distress (Willis et al., 2021). This internal disconnection is compounded by systems that normalize such divisive ideologies.

Internalized white supremacy is embedded in the fabric of our society, making it challenging to identify all of the ways it affects us and our clients. Images about beauty, success, health, productivity, individualism, professional etiquette, and other organizational systems are built upon ideas of white superiority (Jones & Okun, 2001). The mental and emotional injury caused by encounters with racial bias and ethnic discrimination, racism, and hate crimes traumatizes those targeted by such harmful behavior (Helms et al., 2012).

The trauma of internalized racism often spreads through implicit or unconscious biases, known as *microaggressions*. *Microaggressions* are defined as brief and "commonplace daily verbal or behavioral indignities, whether intentional or unintentional, that communicate hostile, derogatory, or negative attitudes toward stigmatized or culturally marginalized groups" (Sue, 2010). When we are a member of the dominant culture and leave our biases unchecked, we knowingly and unknowingly cause harm to people from marginalized populations.

Research has found (Williams, 2020) that microaggressions are commonly found in the therapeutic space, rupturing the therapeutic relationship. Having good intentions is not enough to prevent microaggressions. Microaggressions are imbued with a quality of ambiguity that creates confusion on the part of the target and cover for the perpetrator; therefore, we must actively look within to see where internalized prejudice prevents us from being in full contact with our clients (Lefforge et al., 2019).

Examples of microaggressions include denying an individual as a racial or cultural being; exclusion of literature that represents various racial groups; using a person's culture, which is different from our own, as a Halloween costume; words of encouragement can be microaggressions, such as saying, "I like the way you said that" to a person from a marginalized population, indicating that their tone needs to be palatable to be acceptable.

Internalized racism has been a part of the fabric of society for generations. Racialized trauma is multi-generational, where a person's epigenetics change based on trauma and environmental stressors (Haupt, 2023). Because of this, a client's healing is deeply intertwined with the healing of their ancestral lineage. Interventions that include a client's ancestors offer a transpersonal context in which to work with racialized trauma.

Along with ancestral patterns, somatic interventions support the deeper work of healing racialized trauma (Menakem, 2017). When we work in and through the body, the nervous system can support a client's movement toward a sense of regulation and well-being. When bodily sensations of anger, fear, and hopeless are felt and processed, a client feels more integrated and present. However, some cultures do not feel comfortable working with the body. In these instances, collaborating with our clients for a more top-down way of processing can be useful.

It is an ethical issue in this position of power as a therapist to do the work of anti-racism. We must own the way internalized racism exists within ourselves, and we must create a culture where we can have difficult conversations. We are all affected by internalized ideas about race, and the moment we think we are beyond such prejudices we become at risk of misusing our power. Being an ally isn't enough; we must be a co-conspirator to change systems.

The Therapist's Cultural Lens

With increasing awareness of the way systems of oppression influence our cultural lens, our therapeutic presence becomes more effective. As professionals in the field of mental health, we have an obligation to examine our own thoughts, feelings, and motives as they relate to internalized white supremacy and our cultural lens. Continual self-inquiry as to our own cultural biases is a basic requirement to be ethical and effective.

Understanding that implicit biases live beneath the level of our conscious mind, our somatic intelligence offers us insight into the way we have acquired and perpetuated negative subliminal attitudes toward marginalized populations (Menakem, 2017). Where our thinking brain may hold a story about ourselves as an ally or advocate, our body provides a more honest and uncensored representation of what we have internalized from society.

Being honest with ourselves about our own implicit biases provides us with the integrity needed to be culturally reflexive, where we honor what arises within ourselves when our biases are confronted (Krause, 2012). When we deny our own internalized racism, we are more prone to perpetuate racist ideas (Kendi, 2023). Holding ourselves accountable, especially when we feel discomfort, is integral to the work of social justice. Being with the sensations, vibrations, and emotions in our body will allow us to be with our unconscious prejudices and implicit biases (Menakem, 2017).

Curiosity about our somatic experience is a crucial practice for cultural reflexivity. When we listen to the truth of our biases as expressed through the body, we increase understanding of the way we perceive other people.

Depending on the amount of exposure we have to cultures that vary from our own, we may be caught off-guard when our body reveals our biases. The values, attitudes, and traditions of our cultural group influence our somatic response. When our values are reinforced by the dominant culture, we may unintentionally cause harm when our clients hold extremely different values from our own. When our cultural lens is left unexamined, we may unintentionally speak as if our culture's values were *the* values.

Cultural reflexivity allows us to examine our own lens while staying curious about the lenses, values, attitudes, and traditions of our clients based on their identifying cultural group. Understanding our cultural inheritance makes it possible to stop cycles of harm based on internalized white supremacy. Along with our own cultural reflexivity, we can create a therapeutic container that is welcoming of all cultural and racial identities, as well as being authentically gender-affirming and queer-affirming, with the following considerations:

- ♦ Share our pronouns.
- ♦ Ask our client what their preferred pronouns are.
- ♦ Clarify what certain words, terms, and values mean to them. Even common words and emotions can have different cultural definitions.
- ♦ Discover what is true for our client.
- ♦ Acknowledge cultural differences.
- ♦ Understand our own culture.
- ♦ Engage in self-assessment: How do race, age, ability, gender, gender expression, sexuality, religion, socioeconomic status, size, nationality, status, and language impact the way we move in this world?
- ♦ Acquire cultural knowledge and skills.
- ♦ View behavior within a cultural context.
- ♦ If our clients share ideas that reinforce internalized racism, white supremacy, homophobia, or other negative prejudices, compassionately confront their internalized superiority or inferiority.
- ♦ Work with clients on dismantling what they have internalized.

The Client's Cultural Lens

When we are aware of our own cultural lens, we are less likely to assume that our ideologies are the standard for all people. Aware of the influences on our worldview, we become more open and curious about other people's worldview. Culture influences how individuals experience, perceive, and express mental health symptoms and treatment (Roche & Maxie, 2003). Familiarizing ourselves with different cultures and values offers cultural knowledge and skills to support our clients. In this endeavor, we gain more understanding of the root of their suffering as well as the resources and gifts of their culture.

Barriers of cultural divides are exacerbated when a therapist allows cultural factors and differences to go unacknowledged (Krause, 2012). Our differences are important to see and honor. If we do not talk about cultural lenses and internalized white supremacy, it hinders the therapeutic process and perpetuates internalized white supremacy.

To place culture at the center of our psychotherapy practice is to recognize that individual traits and the environment interact to cause behavior (Krause, 2012). We cannot see a client as separate from their environment, for they exist within a social context. Acknowledging the interaction between a person and their environment is called field theory, and it is a pillar of gestalt therapy (Lewin, 1997). The behaviors and symptoms that our clients experience cannot be seen as detached from the environment.

Recognizing that all clients are affected by internalized white supremacy and systems of oppression, we create a therapeutic container where they can dismantle the ways in which clients organized themselves around the wound of colonization.

When we work with clients who are part of the dominant culture, we must work with them to see the ways in which their own privilege and internalized superiority manifest. When we are in right use of power, the work we do creates a safer and more just society for all. Confronting racism and other forms of misused power when they arise in our therapy room acknowledges that prejudice and discrimination are a mental and behavioral health issue.

Here are some of the differing cultural values and beliefs that we must be aware of in a session:

- ◆ Ideas around health and illness.
- ◆ Mistrust or trust in treatment.
- ◆ Concepts of time and money.
- ◆ Values around collectivism and individualism.
- ◆ Views of spirituality and religion.
- ◆ Beliefs around gender expression and gender roles.
- ◆ Comfort with emotional expression and eye contact.
- ◆ Expression of language usage and parenting styles.

Gender, Sexuality, and Relationship Design

A decolonized approach to healing and transformation is a queering approach to healing and transformation. Gender, gender identity, sexual orientation, and relationship design prejudices are seated in the culture with which we most closely identify (Alman et al., 2023). The polarization of gender as a binary construct is a societal value fueled by patriarchal systems of inequality. These same systems, based on male-centered obsession with dominance and control, influence ideas about sexual orientation and relationship design, where cisgender, heterosexual, monogamous relationships are valued over other expressions of gender identity, sexual identity, and relationship design.

Understanding our own gender identity as societally influenced is paramount in our ability to be with all clients. Cultural assumptions around gender need to be brought into the field of awareness for a client to arrive at full contact with themselves. Instead of assuming a client's gender, we must ask our clients about this sacred expression of their humanity.

Knowing that varying cultures view gender expression differently, we can create space to explore clients' gender development with them.

In the 40 years since homosexuality was removed as a mental illness diagnosis, queer-affirming care has exponentially increased (O'Shaughnessy & Speir, 2018). However, these colonized views are still unknowingly embedded in evidence-based practices, and this is compounded by therapists' internalized homophobia. Relying on a therapist's awareness of their implicit biases has its limitations; however, this self-awareness is needed to create a space for a client to be witnessed in such a way that their humanity is affirmed.

Relationship design refers to the context in which a person chooses to engage romantically. While the dominant culture offers images and messages assuming monogamy will bring satisfaction, consenting adults who choose alternative designs for their relationship are equally satisfied in their relationships (LaSala, 2004). Polyamory, also known as ethical nonmonogamy (ENM), emerges from an honest conversation about intimacy desires. Exploring a range of emotions, from jealousy to compersion (which is joy in seeing one's partner happy), ENM can take many forms. Exploring a client's desires with them can help them to clear societal introjections and expand their capacity for intimacy in whichever relationship design they choose.

When our lens is skewed by internalized societal values, we are more likely to unintentionally cause our clients to feel shame when they do not fit those norms. Our cultural reflexivity is crucial to create a truly safe space for clients to share openly about themselves. It is our ethical duty to look at the way we have been influenced by societal systems so that we don't impose those systems onto our clients.

Nonviolent Space Holding

As we increase awareness of our own cultural lens, we are better able to hold space in a way that is truly nonviolent, where we support our clients' healing without force. Nonviolence is embedded in a therapeutic container where we do not impose our values onto our clients. Instead, we honor our client's culture and racial identity, meeting them at the sacred boundary. We honor their worldview without assuming that they share our perspectives. We see them in their wholeness as we engage with them from our wholeness, trusting that they have the answers to their suffering within them.

Collaboratively co-creating a truly healing space with clients requires that we tend to their patterns of distress with great care. This means that therapeutic interventions are guided by a combination of what our clients want along with our clear observations. Deferring to our clients' autonomy, we follow their wisdom and desire while also guiding them in moving through patterns of distress.

By nature of the therapeutic relationship, the client is granting the therapist a certain authority to guide them through their habitual patterns and unresolved experiences. Building the trust of the therapeutic relationship is ongoing, where the therapist demonstrates their skill and care as provider while also getting a client's consent when offering an intervention.

This reinforces that the client's autonomous will and wisdom are the true guide of the session, and our trained and skillful presence is collaborating with them for their deepest healing.

Another element of building a nonviolent container is through the language we choose when we share a reflection. Our clear witness is an offering for the client to deepen their understanding of themselves. Even when our reflection is not a complete fit for the client, they have the opportunity to clarify for themselves what is deeply true for them. For our witness to be truly nonviolent, our words must signify that what we see is through our perception rather than an ultimate truth about them.

Because there is an inherent power differential that results in a vulnerability on the part of the client, we must ensure that every word we express reinforces the therapeutic culture of nonviolence. Welcoming every aspect of our clients, our nonviolent presence begins to transmute the internalized violence of society. Instead of being another representation of an authority figure who has power *over* them, we co-create *with* them as they reconnect with their authentic power.

Here are some ways to stay client-led and consensual in our work with clients:

♦ Stay connected to our own somatic experiences and be curious about our implicit biases.
♦ Follow the client's energy and meet them where they are.
♦ Gain understanding of what a client is feeling distressed about, and why.
♦ Defer to the client's desire in terms of what they want to change/transform/heal.
♦ Instead of pathologizing the client, stay curious about how they have adapted to systems of oppression not designed for their well-being.
♦ See the wisdom and dignity in the way they learned to survive.
♦ Before trying an intervention or experiment, ask explicitly if the client would like to try something. (We will explore experiments in later chapters.)
♦ Collaborate with the client on how to design the experiment.
♦ Create a therapeutic culture where the client's innate wisdom is the guide for their healing.

Be a Catalyst

We all are impacted by living in a society that is not designed for the well-being of humanity. Systems of oppression maintained by colonized ideas negatively impact all beings, including those who are in positions of privilege (Kendi, 2019). Hierarchies of race, gender, sexuality, ableism, socioeconomic status, and neuro-capabilities perpetuate a society that is out of rhythm with nature.

Engaging with our clients as the expert reinforces the colonized view of mental health and healing. Letting go of our preconceived ideas of what it means to be a therapist, we honor our clients by fully trusting their inherent wisdom. To have our presence, awareness, and energy ignite deep presence, increased awareness, and movement of energy in our clients communicates trust in their process.

When our therapeutic container shines a light on the wound of colonialism, our work begins to dismantle systems of oppression. The inner work in a session has a larger impact in the context of society, as clients influence the environment just as they are influenced by it.

Therapy must be an expression of social justice activism and paradigm shifting. When our awareness is emboldened by the clarity of our own cultural lens, our work becomes a catalyst for healing on a larger scale.

Lessons from the Therapy Room

My location in society as a white cis-woman who is heterosexual, able bodied, and neuro-typical influences my worldview. I was raised in a middle-class family by divorced parents who maintained a good friendship. My mother came from a large Italian Catholic family, and she was a lesbian who was committed to working with survivors of incest. My home was a hub for personal growth workshops, large gatherings, and a safe space for the queer community.

My father was a doctor of osteopathy who came from an Ashkenazi Jewish family. My great-grandfather was a Rabbi in Europe during WWII, and my grandfather immigrated on his own as a teenager and was a women's rights and civil rights activist. My father was a genius physician who was as generous as he was progressive. He was always studying the most holistic, nonviolent forms of medicine and teaching others how to be empowered in their health and healing.

As a child of the 80s, I felt apprehensive about standing out for either my mom's queer identity or my dad's Jewish lineage. Subsequently, I created a persona that would allow me to be as chameleon-like as I could in my suburban Californian town. In spite of my fear of standing out, from a young age, I learned that to be an ally for the LGBTQIA+ (Lesbian, Gay, Bisexual, Transgender, Queer or Questioning, Intersex, and Asexual, and other identities) and BIPOC (Black, Indigenous, People of Color) populations meant to question my own privilege. Although my cultural lens was that of the dominant culture, I was aware that the default settings of this culture were not designed for the health and well-being of all people. To be in integrity with the values I learned from my parents, I needed to question my own assumptions and challenge the assumptions of those from the dominant culture.

In my work with clients, my awareness of my own cultural lens and my clients' cultural lenses is always in my field of awareness. When I am sitting with any client, I consciously question my own assumptions and biases to ensure that I do not perpetuate patterns of harm as a member of the dominant culture. I also stay curious about my client's assumptions and biases to discover what internalized beliefs perpetuate systems of oppression.

I recall a time when I was sitting with a client who was a white heterosexual cis-woman, upper middle-class, able bodied, and neuro-typical. She arrived to her session feeling distraught by feedback she had recently gotten from her boyfriend and her best friend. Both of them had told her that she was self-centered and hard to talk to. She had tears in her eyes and was visibly shaken by these remarks, and she wanted to be self-reflexive and look within to see if what they said might have some truth.

She began by telling me that her friend, who was a member of the BIPOC community, told my client that she didn't feel safe around her. She told her that she felt marginalized in her presence, and she was upset at various ways my client dismissed her invitations to be an ally. She shared that she didn't feel safe around my client, and she called my client a racist.

My client was indignant: "I'm not a racist. She's the racist. She's saying that because I'm white, I'm bad. This is reverse racism!"

"I see you're upset," I said. "As I hear your story, I want to teach you some things about racism and anti-racism. Are you open to that?"

She eagerly agreed, stating that she wanted to learn and hear what I had to say. "Reverse racism does not exist. As long as systems of oppression exist at the level of society, there cannot be reverse racism."

"But I don't see color!" she exclaimed. "And besides, she's the privileged one. She comes from money and her parents help her out."

"Privilege, in this case, has nothing to do with money or wealthy parents. We are talking about racism and internalized white supremacy. You said you want to reflect on what she said about you, but you seem defensive."

"I just don't understand. I have Black friends. I'm not a racist."

"There is no such thing as 'not being a racist.' You are either racist or you are anti-racist, working as an ally to dismantle systems of oppression."

"She told me that she went up to a Black woman at a work function and asked her if she felt safe because everyone else was white. That's racist! I'm not racist!"

"It sounds like she was being an ally to someone who was marginalized. Allyship and anti-racism require that we acknowledge racial identities and act to create safe spaces for marginalized individuals."

"But she's the racist. She's the one singling people out because of their race!"

"You seem defensive. Let's pause for a moment. Where do you feel that in your body?"

"Everywhere."

"Take a few breaths and feel that defensiveness is everywhere." After a few moments of silent breathing, I said, "Now look within to see who you are defending and why."

"I don't want to be seen as bad. I want her to see that she is bad so she'll see I'm good."

"Just notice you want to be seen as good. Take a few breaths and let yourself feel that. In the past few years, there has been a paradigm shift in our understanding of racism and anti-racism, so these concepts might be new to you. I think your friend has pointed to something within yourself that is essential for you to look at."

After the session ended, I gave my client some resources to learn more about being an anti-racist. She texted me later thanking me, saying she had found her way back to humility and compassion.

I share this example with you to highlight that this is my ethical duty as a therapist. I must actively confront racism when I see it, and these moments may not seem client-led. However, to be in right use of power, I must take a stand against harmful societal values that keep people in marginalized groups oppressed. And it is my deep honor to do so.

Exercise: Explore Your Location in Society

- Age
- Socioeconomic status
- Gender
- Gender expression
- Sexual orientation
- Size
- Nationality
- Language
- Race
- Religion
- Physical ability
- Mental ability

How do your social locations impact the way you move in this world? Are there identities of privilege? Identities of oppression? Where do they intersect? How might this introspection help you show up as an anti-racist therapist?

References

Alman, G., & Kolmannskog, V. (2023). *Queering gestalt therapy: An anthology on gender, sex, and relationship diversity in psychotherapy.* Routledge.

Haupt, L. (2023). *Rooted: Life at the crossroads of science, nature, and spirit.* Little, Brown Spark.

Helms, N., Nicolas, G., & Green, C. E. (2012). *Racism and ethnoviolence as trauma: Enhancing professional training.* Sage Journals.

Jones, K., & Okun, T. (2001). *Dismantling racism: A workbook for social change groups.* ChangeWork.

Kendi, I. (2019). *How to be an antiracist.* One World Publishers

Kendi, I. (2023). *How to Be an Antiracist.* Updated edition. One World.

Krause, I. B. (2012). *Culture and reflexivity in systemic psychotherapy: Mutual perspectives.* Routledge.

LaSala, M. C. (2004). Extradyadic sex and gay male couples: Comparing monogamous and nonmonogamous relationships. Families in society. *The Journal of Contemporary Social Services, 85*(3), 405–412.

Lefforge, N., McLaughlin, S., & Goats-Jones, M. (2019). A training model for addressing microaggressions in group psychotherapy. *International Journal of Group Psychotherapy, 70*(1), 1–28.

Lewin, K. (1997). *Resolving social conflicts and field theory in social science.* American Psychological Association.

Menakem, R. (2017). *My grandmother's hands: Racialized trauma and the pathway to mending our hearts and bodies.* Las Vegas: Central Recovery Press.

Mullan, J. (2023). *Decolonizing therapy: Oppression, historical trauma, and politicizing your practice.* W.W. Norton.

O'Shaughnessy, T., & Speir, Z. (2018). The state of LGBQ affirmative therapy clinical research: A mixed-methods systematic synthesis. *Psychology of Sexual Orientation and Gender Diversity, 5*(1), 82–98.

Perls, F. (1978). *The Gestalt approach and eye-witness to therapy.* Bantam Books.

Perls, F. (1992). *Gestalt therapy verbatim* (2nd ed.). The Gestalt Journal Press.

Perls, F., Hefferline, R., & Goodman, P. (1951). *Gestalt therapy: Excitement and growth in the human personality.* The Gestalt Journal Press.

Pyke, K. (2010). What is internalized racial oppression and why don't we study it? Acknowledging racism's hidden injuries. Sociological Perspectives, 53(4), 551–572.

Roche, M., & Moxie, A. (2003). Ten considerations in addressing cultural differences in psychotherapy. *Professional Psychology: Research and Practice, 34*(2), 180–186.

Sue, D. W. (2010). *Macroaggressions: More than just race.* Psychology Today.

Williams, M. (2020). *Managing microaggressions: Addressing everyday racism in therapeutic spaces.* Oxford University Press.

Willis, H., Sosoo, E., & Neblett, E. (2021). *The associations between internalized racism, racial identity, and psychological distress* (Vol. 9, No. 2). Sage Journals.

Chapter 4

Spirituality and Subtle Energy

Psychological healing is not separate from spirituality, for humanity cannot be reduced down to separate and detached parts. Spirituality and metaphysics are elements of the whole *gestalt*, where the essence of a client's spiritual nature is interconnected with their psychological state. Spontaneity and naturalness are the primary virtues of innate spirituality (Miller, 2022). When a therapist places a framework onto a client, they are at risk of interrupting the natural flow and spontaneity of the client's Source of healing. It is the task of the therapist to engage in the therapeutic relationship in ways that allow nature to guide the client's healing and transformation (Brownell, 2010).

When we access higher levels of awareness in the therapy room, we allow the relational field to become a foundation for higher spiritual development for both ourselves and our clients (Lynn, 2006). Our awareness expands, and our spiritual alignment flows synergistically with our clients. As we become more aware and aligned in our clients' presence, they also become more aware and aligned as they move through the session. By honoring the naturalistic, metaphysical, and anti-authoritarian ethos built into gestalt theory, spirituality becomes the organic catalyst that allows for integration, healing, and transformation to manifest within the client (Brownell, 2010).

The ancient wisdom of Zen Buddhism and Taoism is the basis for this mindfulness-based, nonviolent approach to counseling (Shonin & Van Gordon, 2014; Dahlsgaard et al., 2005). The Buddhist teaching of the *eightfold path* offers us a philosophy of what unfolds as a client returns to the true nature of their innate spirituality.

The eightfold path relates to psychotherapy as follows (Naranjo, 1978): Through the clinician's clear witness, the client moves from confusion to understanding and gains a *right view* of reality. As they become more aware and compassionate with themselves, resistance and clinging transmute into understanding and harmlessness with *right resolve*. From this place, they see the harm caused by deceitful and divisive speaking and learn to cultivate *right speech*. This same intention is brought into behavior, where a person abstains from self-betrayal and harmful deeds with *right action*. With their ego no longer the driving force of their existence, they engage in *right livelihood* where shared resources supersede capitalism. The energy they put forth in their life comes from innocence and wholesomeness, cultivating *right effort*. Ongoing practice of tending to their state of mind through therapy and meditation creates *right mindfulness*. All of this supports the integration and unification of *right Samadhi* or equanimity, where clients begin to move through the world with calmness and level-headedness.

DOI: 10.4324/9781003521969-5

When we participate in a session in such a way that a client's innate spirituality guides their transformation, this noble path to enlightenment is the natural outcome. We must be aware not to offer any spiritual ideology to the client, for we run the risk of becoming another voice of *should* in their world and bypass therapeutic opportunities. We neither ignore nor lead a client in spiritual or religious ideology. Instead, we allow Spirit to be our co-therapist as we open to transcendent and mystical realms that offer insight and guidance to the process of integration. Clients organically find their way to living in alignment with their true nature.

Honoring Subtle Energy

One way that innate spirituality can be accessed in the therapy room is through attunement to *subtle energy.* Subtle energy is the expression of a person's vital force. This energy moves up through the midline of the body and corresponds with vital organs and nerves. From the midline of the body, vitality emanates outward, creating an energy field around the physical body. Research has found that the heart, for example, emits an electromagnetic field that changes based on our emotions (McCraty et al., 1995). This same research found that other people can sense the quality of our emotions through the electromagnetic energy that radiates from our heart. The subtle energy of the electromagnetic field can actually be measured several feet away from the body.

The expression of a client's state of being manifests through their subtle energy. When their inner state is characterized by spiritual alignment and mindfulness, a client's energy body is more likely to express as supple and clear. When their inner state is characterized by unprocessed emotions and rigid thought patterns, a client's energy body is restricted, dense, and thwarted. Gaining clarity about emotions and thoughts is an essential component of making room for the wholeness of the client. As we do this, we also have an opportunity to bring attention to the more subtle elements of their lived experience, for these are the spiritual threads where innate wisdom guides them through their experience and back home to themselves.

Attuning to subtle energy is akin to attuning to the air quality: When the air seems fresh, it looks and feels differently than when it seems polluted. Because unprocessed emotions and experiences living within a client's subtle energy body look and feel similar to the air quality, this is frequently referred to as *emotional energy pollution* (EEP) (Orr, 2013). EEP has the appearance of a vaporous muck within a person's energy body that veils the full expression of their spiritual Self. It is also possible to see and sense the absence of EEP, where the subtle energy body is clear and iridescent.

One way to conceptualize EEP is throughthe analogy of a seedy bar. A seedy bar is a place where people get blackout drunk, have violent outbursts, drug others, and suppress their own vitality. Walking into a seedy bar, we may be able to see the thick, vaporous residue of the EEP that resides there. We may feel unpleasant in this space, like we can't quite relax or take a deep breath. This *psychic dirt* is a discharge of the energy of the people who frequent this place.

This analogy can be compared to one of a retreat center. A retreat center is a place where people engage in devotional practices and dedicate their mind, heart, and energy to spiritual evolution. For this example, everyone at the retreat center, including those in leadership, steward the land, honor their bodies as sacred, and treat one another with reverence. Although some sacred spaces have a misuse of power, in this example, all beings are honored and empowered at this retreat center. Walking into this space, we may be able to see and sense the vibrant clarity of the energy of this space. We may take a deep breath and feel more relaxed here. The purity of this energy is a reflection of the way those present listen to and honor the information offered from their EEP.

This same example can be applied to people: Those who suppress their vitality, accumulate unfinished business, and/or engage in self-sabotage store more EEP in their system than those who inspire their vitality, resolve unfinished business, and engage in life-affirming behaviors. Although all of us have expereinces that create EEP, how we tend to ourselves is what informs the degree of clarity in our system.

Depending on our sensitivity and attunement, we can see and sense EEP in the subtle energy body of our clients visually, intuitively, and physically. However, our ability to see EEP is not necessary in order to honor subtle energy. As a client talks about themselves, we invite them to attune to their inner mind–body connection. In these moments, they may feel EEP through sensations of stuckness and heaviness. When we bring our attention to the stuckness and invite the client to stay present to the sensation, it becomes the entry point to transmuting what has been previously undigested. Discovering what it's holding and what it needs is the way we honor subtle energy as part of the client's wholeness.

Another way to attune to a client's EEP is by sensing it in our own body. Feeling a client's stored emotional energy in our body is often the first presentation of intuitively witnessing subtle energy. Tension in our solar plexus, heaviness in our heart, tightness around our throat, or some other sensation that clearly is not our own offers insight into where EEP is being held. Attuning to our own experience in these moments and honoring this sensation allows it to become useful to the therapeutic process. Instead of sharing that we are having a sensation, we can use this information to ask our clients what they feel in this place within their own being.

Some of us may be able to see the subtle energy of the client with our metaphysical eyes. Hazy or dark residue within and around the client's body can be seen throughout a session. With this degree of attunement, we can also see when it moves and their energy becomes clarified. When we have this capacity, we hold our seeing loosely and use it to direct attention to certain areas of the client's being. We may ask them what they notice in this particular part of their body, or we may let them know how they seem to us. For example, "It seems like your heart is holding something. What do you notice there?" In this way, we honor both ourselves and the client in the subtle realm.

When we listen to and follow subtle energy, our clients begin to see within themselves what has been blocking their connection to their spiritual essence. This makes it more possible for them to process past events and regulate their nervous system. Honoring the information of their subtle energy allows them a way to find their way back home to their true nature.

Anatomy of the Energy Body

Attuning to our clients' subtle energy body does not require that we know the anatomy of the energy body. Staying infinitely curious and open to intuitive wisdom is more important than learning a map. This is, in part, what makes this work nonviolent. A client's account of what is being held in any area of the physical body and subtle energy is more valuable information than putting our understanding of subtle energy onto our clients. Learning about the energy body, however, is supportive in understanding the ways that EEP inhibits a client's sense of well-being. The energy body stores the consciousness of unfinished business, stress, and pain. As we gain understanding of the way a client's psychological state is housed in their energy body, we begin to see the importance of subtle energy in mental health healing.

There are seven energetic focal points or centers up the midline of the body, called *chakras*. Above the head there are 3 lesser-known chakras, and below the base of the spine there are 2 more, making 12 total up the midline of the body. Beyond the midline of the body, there are 114 chakras in total, spreading throughout the etheric subtle body (Judith, 2015).

Since the seven energy focal points up the midline of the body often correlate with sensations, the client's awareness can easily perceive them. These energy centers have been found to communicate with the brain through the transmission of nerve impulses, neurotransmitters, hormones, and energetically through electromagnetic field interactions (McCraty, 2015). Around the physical body, there are five layers of our energy body that express the state of our inner energy layers.

When we bring awareness to subtle energy blocks, we support the awakening of the subtle body and the integration of the inner mind–body experience. When EEP is cleared, vital energy flows naturally and spontaneously up the midline of the body. This is where a client's spiritual alignment emerges in connection with an overall sense of well-being. The fuller expression of their energy body is one of health, where their vital force supports toned energetic boundaries.

What follows is the anatomy of the seven energy focal points up the midline of the body, as well as the five energetic layers around the body (Dale, 2009) (Figure 4.1). The general experience of an open energy center and a blocked energy center is also described. Because these energy centers are generalizable to all people, they are explored from a collective lens, where both the therapist and the client (we) have these energy centers:

1. **Root:** The root chakra is located at the base of the spine, and it houses our sense of stability and safety.
   - When the root is open, we seat ourselves in the foundation of self-trust and inner stability.
   - When the root is closed, we feel unsafe in life, and we are disconnected from our solid, inner foundation. Because of this, we look to others for our sense of safety and stability.
2. **Sacral:** The sacral chakra is located just below the belly button and houses the energy of our creativity and sexuality.

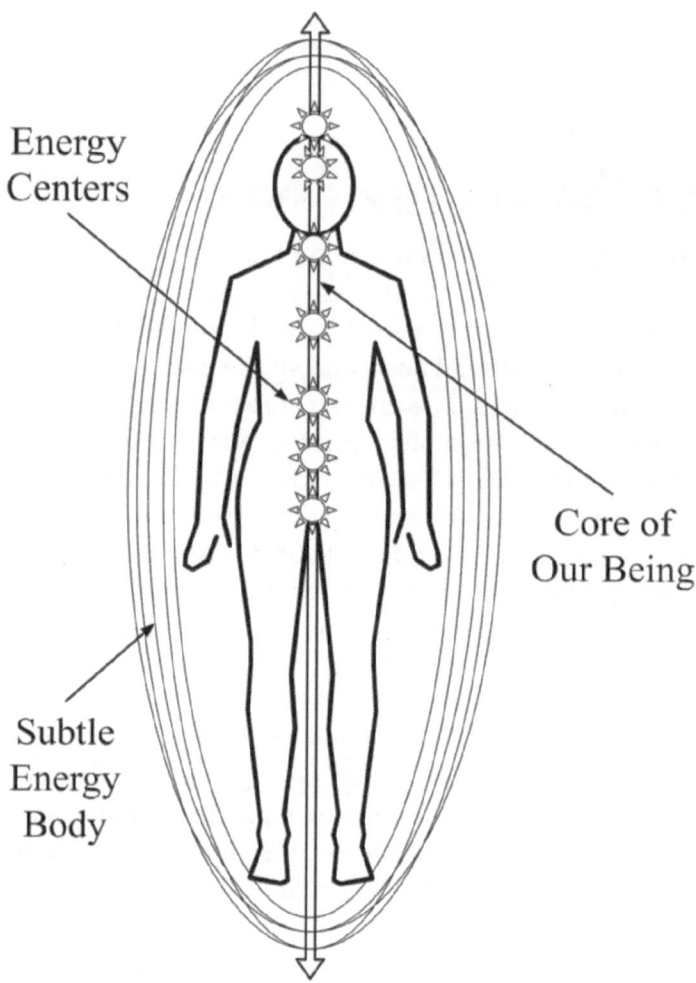

Energy
Centers

Core of
Our Being

Subtle
Energy
Body

Figure 4.1 Subtle Energy Body (Kwiker, 2022, p. 91)

- ○ When the sacral chakra is open, we explore the pleasure and bliss of being in a body. Creative transmissions express through us with ease, and we feel pleasure as we create.
- ○ When the sacral chakra is blocked, we are storing unprocessed fear and staying self-protected in creativity and sexual intimacy.
3. **Solar Plexus:** The solar plexus is located near the diaphragm, about 3–4 inches above the belly button. It houses the energy of our confidence and congruence, where our own will is expressed through action.
- ○ When the solar plexus is open, we are in right action, where what we think, say, and do is congruent with the truth of who we are.
- ○ When the solar plexus is blocked, our actions are not congruent with the truth of who we are. Our self-esteem and confidence are hidden by shame, and we give our will over to others.
4. **Heart:** The heart center is located in the center of our chest, right at our sternum. It houses the energy of our love and compassion.
- ○ When the heart center is open, we are compassionate and loving, with healthy boundaries based on our values, not our reactions.
- ○ When the heart center is closed, we are self-protected, resentful, and orient to-wards grief.

5. **Throat:** The throat center is located in our throat, and it houses the energy of our communication. Emotional expressions, as well as being honest and authentic with our thoughts, desires, and creativity, are stored here.
    o When the throat center is open, we use our authentic voice with words and sounds. We own our emotions and communicate on behalf of what we value.
    o When the throat center is blocked, we complain, withhold our emotions, and have difficulty saying what's true for us.
6. **Third Eye:** Located between the eyes, this center houses our access to our inner knowing and creative imagination.
    o When the third eye is open, intuitive transmissions enter clearly into our awareness. We can see infinite possibilities for ourselves, and we trust ourselves to make decisions in service of the highest good.
    o When this center is blocked, we are disconnected from our deeper knowing and intuition. We look to other people for the answer, not trusting ourselves, and anticipating the worst-case scenario. We expect bad things to happen, and we worry about what thatmight be.
7. **Crown:** Located at the top of the head, this center represents our spiritual connection.
    o When the crown is open, we can easily sense our innate spiritual Self, our interconnectedness with universal wisdom, and our divine wholeness.
    o When the crown is closed, we feel disconnected from our spiritual Self; we cling to our thought-based ego identity and perceive spirituality and divinity as something outside of ourselves.

Aside from the energy focal points up the midline of the body, we also have energetic layers around our body, called *kushas* (Dale, 2009). These energetic layers measure up to several feet away from the body and express our mental, physical, and emotional health and clarity.

Beginning from the outside in, here are the five layers of the energy body:

1. **Physical Layer:** Located closest to the dense energy of our human form, this layer represents physical well-being and health.
    o When we are vital and healthy, the physical layer of our energy body is both soft and strong.
    o When our vitality is deficient and/or when we cling to our human form as our identity, the physical layer of our energy body is deflated and dense.
2. **Life Force Layer:** The life force layer is the second layer of our energy body, located just beyond our physical layer. It is responsible for the expression of our vitality and connection to all of life.
    o When the life force layer is healthy, we flow with the natural rhythm of nature, and our energy is fluid.
    o When the life force layer is depleted, we feel and act more rigid as we try to conserve our energy.
3. **Mental Layer:** The mental layer is the third layer, which is responsible for our access to thinking and seeing clearly.
    o When the mental layer is clear, our mind is clear, and our energy responds with similar clarity.
    o When our mental layer is blocked, our mind is jumbled or confused.

4. **Wisdom Layer:** As the fourth layer of our energy body, the wisdom layer holds our intuition.
    ○ When our wisdom layer is clear, we fully trust our wise, mature Self and our intuitive senses.
    ○ When our wisdom layer is blocked, we ignore our intuition and look to others for the answers.
5. **Bliss Body:** Located the furthest from our physical body, the bliss body is the deepest and most subtle layer of the energy body. This is where bliss, our original state, resides.
    ○ When our bliss body is clear, we open to pleasure without working to experience bliss or joy.
    ○ When our bliss body is blocked, we put in effort to find pleasure and inhibit the softness of our bliss. Figure 4.1

Blocked Subtle Energy

When a client's energetic focal points are open and clear, their vital force moves freely in alignment with the core of their being. This is the center of their vital force, which holds the boundless energy of life itself. From this place of alignment, the client is fully present and in contact with their spiritual nature. They feel a sense of inner peace and joy, and their body is relaxed. They recognize their life as meaningful, and they perceive the interconnectedness of all of life.

Blocked energy holds the residue of unprocessed experiences. Attuning to subtle energy reveals the energetic holding patterns that correlate with the client's psychological, behavioral, emotional, and physical patterns. As we contact energetic holding patterns, we must not try to change them or qualify them as *bad*. It's simply therapeutic material that informs the client's process as they move through what they have been storing.

When these energetic focal points are thwarted by unprocessed emotions and experiences, vital force is distorted, and the person feels off center from the core of their being. The person often clings to their mind and disowns a deeper truth within themselves. This is known as the top-dog/under-dog dynamic, where an inner conflict manifests in order to avoid a conflict with the environment (Perls et al., 1951). The top-dog often houses a person's *shouldism*, and the under-dog holds the truth of the person's desires.

The top-dog/under-dog dynamic holds the energy of an inner polarity, where there are two opposing constructs seemingly at odds with one another. This polarity is expressed as two points of blocked energy, causing the subtle energy body to be thwarted. In Figure 4.2, we can see the way a person's vital force is thwarted by this inner conflict. When they are identified with their thought-based reality and disowning their shadow, a distortion in their energy body manifests.

Figure 1.3. The image shows a person depicting the line of distortion, with a mask to the left of their head and a shadow of themselves to the right of their foot; a wavy line from the mask to the shadow illustrates their distorted life force energy (Kwiker, 2022).

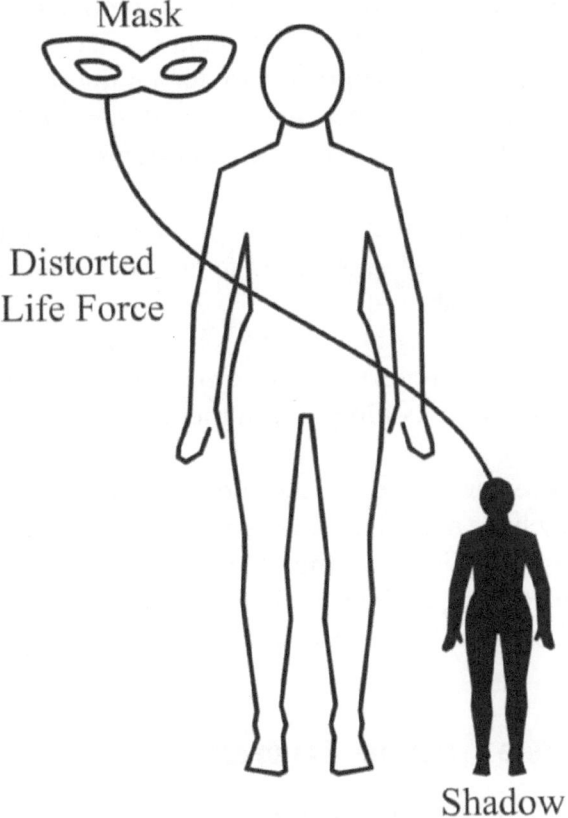

Mask

Distorted
Life Force

Shadow

Figure 4.2 Line of Distortion (Kwiker, 2022, p. 79)

When clients see themselves and their environment through distorted life force energy, their words and energy are filtered through wounds from the past. Energetically, this may appear as a veil skewing their perception and warping their clarity. This mistunement is experienced in their physical, emotional, mental, and spiritual bodies. When we attune to the mistunement of our client's energy, we can support our clients in cultivating energetic coherence, where they experience a sense of "harmonious order, connectedness, stability and efficient use of energy" (McCraty, 2015).

Below is a list of how the seven energy focal points may show up in sessions when they are blocked:

1. **Root:** When this center is blocked, either the client cannot feel their perineum or they clench it tightly. They tend to look to other people for their source of security and safety, and they do not trust themselves to stay seated within their inner foundation of Self. They tend not to honor themselves in relationships, and they do this to try to find connection and safety in others as opposed to within themselves.

2. **Sacral:** When this center is blocked, the client typically reports feeling numbness or a pit in their stomach. Holding on to fear related to their worthiness blocks their creative thinking, and they tend to check out as opposed to turning on their creative expression or sensuality.

3. **Solar Plexus:** When this center is blocked, the client typically feels either emptiness or constriction in their solar plexus, as if there were a rubber band around their diaphragm. The client typically has patterns of self-betrayal, where their actions are not congruent with their deepest desire and truth.

4. **Heart:** When this center is blocked, the client is hunched over and appears self-protected or guarded. Their breath is often heavy with grief, and they can be antagonistic with themselves as opposed to displaying self-compassion. They can also be resentful toward others and personalize the way others treat them.

5. **Throat:** When this center is blocked, the client often reports feelings of a ball in their throat or like they are being strangled. They may appear to cap their emotions off in their throat, and either they are quiet or they want to scream. They tend to blame others for their feelings as opposed to honoring their emotions and their truth with self-responsibility.

6. **Third Eye:** When this center is blocked, the client will often furrow their brow and appear worried. They may report feeling confused or lost, and they may look to us for advice as opposed to looking within themselves for their Source of intuitive wisdom.

7. **Crown:** When this center is blocked, the client's energy is often condensed in their head, and they may have a headache. When asked what they notice in their body, they will likely respond with what they are thinking. The client will talk about the people in their life, looking to them as their Source of love and worth as opposed to connecting with their own innate divinity within themselves.

Five Ways to Move Subtle Energy

Without access to elevated awareness, clients continue to organize themselves around habitual patterns of stored energy. When we think that we are seeing a subtle energy pattern in the client, it is important that we name what we are seeing in a way that *owns our perception as our own* and *collaborates with what is true for the client.* In this way, we meet the client at the sacred boundary, where our clear reflection interacts with their perception. This allows them to activate subtle and awake awareness, which are the most vital resources in clearing stored emotional energy from the subtle body.

Maintaining a neutral presence, we do not qualify certain sensations, thoughts, and emotions as either good or bad—they are simply what is here right now. From the in-between dimension of the I–Thou, we have the capacity to be with the subtle energy blocks from our own awake awareness. This amplifies the client's access to their energy and makes the mobilizing of the energy more potent. Through our invitations, clients are offered a space to become more present and more mindful with what is within them in this moment. Once they are aware of their subtle energy holding pattern, we can invite them to listen for what it needs to mobilize.

Here are five ways we can support the movement of our client's subtle energy:

1. **Awareness:** Awareness mobilizes stored emotional energy, similarly to stirring up dust. Wrapping a session or thought with loving, awake awareness creates an opening in the energy body. Being with their energy consciously, clients learn from their energy and discover what it needs to be resolved.

2. **Breath:** Breath is the only part of the autonomic nervous system that we have conscious control over, and it is essential in regulation. Breath also ignites vital force, and when we tap into the wisdom of the breath, a client can clarify and move stored energy.

3. **Tone:** Listening to an energy block and giving it a voice can be so helpful in supporting its movement. Either words or a simple sound that matches what is being held can move subtle energy. For example, "If your heart had a voice, what would it say?" or "If you'd like, give the sensation in your throat a tone. I want to hear what it has to say" are invitations that support the natural unblocking of stored energy.

4. **Touch:** When a client touches the part of the body that corresponds with their subtle energy holding pattern, they can self-soothe and clear their energy. Massaging their third eye or placing a hand on the heart can be the compassionate awareness they need from themselves to move the energy.

5. **Movement:** Listening to the body, and allowing the energy to unwind in a way that feels natural and loving, can support the movement of subtle energy. Scooping the energy up and flicking it with the hands sometimes occurs spontaneously when a client sees what they've been holding. Rocking the body or twisting happens, or even standing up and shaking off the energy can occur spontaneously to move energy.

As clients become aware of the sensations in their body, they look at the sensations from ordinary awareness. With our support, they learn to attune to their subtle energy and shift into subtle awareness. From this place, they shine the awareness of their mind onto the sensation.

For example, from the mind, they might look down at their root chakra and know that they cannot feel their root. As they shift to subtle awareness, they sense into the absence of feeling and discover that their root is closed. Moving into awake awareness, they enter into the consciousness of the energy in the root, not from the mind but from awareness itself. They experience the root fully, and naturally enter into their phenomenology. From this present moment experience, they reconnect with their root, and their energy begins to flow spontaneously. This is the doorway into their spiritual nature.

When all of the energy focal points clear, clients reconnect with their spiritual alignment. The naturalness and spontaneity of their True Self re-emerge as the general sense of being well and vitality is restored. The subtle energy body around the physical body responds by getting clearer, fuller, and fluffier, and the client can discover how they want to be with themselves and their environment from their most awake, resourced Self.

From their alignment, therapy becomes a place where the elements of the eightfold path are clarified. *Right view* of reality, *right resolve, right speech, right action, right livelihood, right effort, right mindfulness,* and *right Samadhi* unfold from their spiritual connection along with therapeutic inquiry. When a client's thoughts, words, feelings, and actions are congruent with their spiritual Self, their alignment expresses through them in all areas of life. This sacred work is the natural unfolding of a client's health as it is directed by their deepest wisdom.

Lessons from the Therapy Room

As my own spiritual development progressed, my work with clients became more potent. I became more seated in my Self as a clinician, and my presence was a catalyst for clients to return to their true nature. I had been honoring my abilities to see subtle energy, which opened my access to other clairsenses. Along with seeing subtle energy, I began to hear, sense, know, smell, and taste intuitive transitions.

As I sat with a client, they shared with me the thoughts that were swirling around in their mind, and I invited them into direct experience with their swirling thoughts. The moment I offered this invitation, the client became acutely aware of what they really wanted. This desire was at odds with their thought-based reality.

I witnessed my client's inner conflict with my metaphysical eyes, and I saw their distorted life force. Across their face, diagonally from one side of their body to the other, their energy appeared warped. Because this was a new experience, I was unsure what this intuition was offering.

Over the course of that week, each client I saw had an energetic expression of distorted life force. I brought this insight into my contemplative practice, and I meditated on the distortion. Toward the end of my practice, I realized what was being revealed to me: Clinging to the mask of their personality while pushing their truth into the shadow caused their vitality to twist.

I drew my vision on a piece of paper, and I continued to contemplate how to use this information in my work with clients. Over the next few weeks, I practiced following the distorted energy to discover what it was holding. I started listening to the energy to hear what it needed to be resolved, and clients began to open to themselves in new and surprising ways. Once their energy was no longer bound up, the gestalt experiments we did together were much more effective.

Clients described feeling more like themselves than they ever remembered feeling. Many had experience of flow states, where they were in harmony with the energy of the universe. The spiritual experience of timelessness and expressions of creativity emerged, as well as a general sense of well-being.

Exercise: Attuning to Subtle Energy

For this exercise, you will practice giving voice to your attunement to the subtle. Find a partner and set the timer for 10 min. In that time, you will only use subtle energy attunement with language that holds what you're seeing loosely. As you practice with your partner, discover the language that fits for you and notice how it lands with the client.

Examples of subtle attunement include, "You seem open," or "It seems like you're holding a lot in your shoulders," or "Your breath seems to stop at your heart."

Sentence stems to try include, "You seem ..." "It seems ...," "I think I'm sensing ...."

A note on neurodivergence: When a client is neurodivergent, they may feel extremely uncomfortable with this level of attunement. Using this attunement to honor the client and what they need can be supportive to their healing. For example, "You seem uncomfortable." If this is true for the client, offer to try an experiment where you close your eyes or turn away. Doing this in a contactful way supports the client in feeling welcomed as they are.

References

Brownell, P. (2010). Spirituality in the praxis of gestalt therapy. In J. H. Ellens (Ed.), *The healing power of spirituality: How faith helps humans thrive* (Vol. 3), pp. 2–26.

Dahlsgaard, K., Peterson, C., & Seligman, M. (2005)-. Shared virtue: The convergence of valued human strengths across culture and history. *Review of General Psychology, 9*(3), 201–213.

Dale, C. (2009). *The subtle body: An encyclopedia of your energetic anatomy.* Sounds True.

Judith, A. (2015). *Anodea Judith's chakra yoga.* Llewellyn Publications.

Kwiker, H. (2022). *Align: Living and loving from the true self.* Mantra Books.

Lynn, W. (2006). Spirituality and gestalt: A gestalt-transpersonal perspective. *Gestalt Review, 10*(1), 6–21.

McCraty, R. (2015). *The science of the heart* (1st ed.). HeartMath.

McCraty, R., Atkinson, M., Tiller, W. A. Rein, G., & Watkins, A. D. (1995). The effects of emotions on short-term power spectrum analysis of heart rate variability. *The American Journal of Cardiology, 76*(14), 1089–1093.

Miller, L. (2022). *The Awakened Brain: The Psychology of Spirituality.* Penguin Books Ltd. 1st edition.

Naranjo, C. (1978). Gestalt therapy as a transpersonal approach. *Gestalt Journal, 1*(2), 75–81.

Orr, L. (2013). *Haidakhan Babaji Speaks.* Hara Press.

Perls, F., Hefferline, R., & Goodman, P. (1951). *Gestalt therapy: Excitement and growth in the human personality.* Souvenir Press.

Shonin, E., & Van Gordon, W. (2014). The emerging role of buddhism in clinical psychology: Toward effective integration: Psychology of religion and spirituality. *American Psychological Association, 6*(2), 123–137.

Chapter 5

Skills for Holding a Sacred Container

When a therapeutic container is created from our spiritual devotion, we create a sacred space for clients to return to their true nature. Every aspect of our work as a psychotherapist becomes a spiritual practice when we stay aligned and connected with our Self. By being present in the here and now, we welcome everything about a client. Our level of awareness is vital in this practice, as this supports our ability to hold space from our awareness-based knowing.

In ordinary awareness, we perceive clients as a separate other. From this state of consciousness, our words tend to create more disconnection and invite clients to retreat to their minds. The same words offered from a deeper place within ourselves can create more spaciousness, more awareness, and more self-responsibility. The practice of letting go of our thoughts as we sit with a client allows us to explore the meditative quality of a holding space from an awakened state.

We may arrive to a session with our awareness seated in our thinking mind. As we meet our client in the here and now, our awareness naturally expands. From ordinary awareness, we enter into direct experience and sense within ourselves and our clients a subtle energy that is not perceivable from our thought-based reality. Attuning to the more subtle aspects of what is present, we cultivate a relationship with the sacred nature of the therapeutic relationship. When our wisdom interacts with our clients' wisdom, therapy can become a mystical experience that is beyond the logic of any analysis or interpretation.

When our space holding is a sacred offering, our expansive presence is both solid and infinite. As the container of Mother Earth holds the client at every step on their sacred journey, we can invite them to become more present with this infinite resource holding them always. Honoring the ever-present sacred container of Mother Earth supports the container we hold with our awareness and presence.

The container is set through our intentional and devotional space holding, and this sacred practice is reinforced with the words we speak. What follows are the foundational skills for holding a sacred container, as well as the intuitive transmission that may come forth from this place of reverence. Because the foundations of space holding are essential to everything that unfolds in a session, they are worthy of revisiting often. Consider the metaphor of learning to dance: The new dancer wants to do the big moves, but the advanced dancer knows that the basic steps are what make those big moves possible. Attuned communication skills make the more advanced interventions possible.

DOI: 10.4324/9781003521969-6

SevenSkills for Empathetic Listening

Empathetic listening is an active listening that emphasizes hearing the deeper emotions and needs beneath the narratives. The listener responds with reflections that are attuned expressions of understanding what is being conveyed by the speaker, both intellectually and emotionally (Rosenberg, 2015).

When we reflect, if we do so not from our mind but from our awareness, our reflections serve several purposes: We become present with the client, as the words they just said are now being said by us. We contact the client where they are, as we are not interpreting their words when we reflect them. We are keeping the energy of the container clear and clean, as we are giving them their words back to them. We are confirming that we understand them, as we are not assuming that we heard them accurately. We are processing their words through our awareness and giving their words back to them imbued with the light of awareness.

1. **Word-for-Word Reflections:** Saying the client's own words back to them, imbued with awareness and compassion.
2. **Paraphrasing:** Rephrasing what the client just said in your own words, illuminating their narratives with awake awareness.
3. **Key-Word Quoting:** When a client says one word or phrase that seems important or unique to them, reflect that one word or phrase to highlight it with awareness.
4. **Mapping:** Summarizing what's been said over time, stating the main ideas they've expressed that are the most poignant aspects of the narrative, illuminating how they are part of an interconnected whole (more on this later).
5. **Compassionate Listening:** Reflecting the deeper need beneath what's been said: "It sounds like you want …."
6. **Deep Listening:** Reflecting the deeper meaning of what's been said while rephrasing it in your own words: "I think I'm hearing this as …."
7. **Making a guess at their why:** Without analyzing the client, we can offer a reflection that brings their deeper *why* to the awareness field though our guess: "Am I hearing this as...?"

Five Skills for Empathetic Witnessing

Empathetic witnessing is an active observing that emphasizes seeing *how* the client expresses, rather than *what* they say.. The witness offers reflections that are attuned and neutral observations, which communicate a non-judgmental, compassionate reflection.

1. **Seeing Their Expression:** Bringing their physical and emotional expression to the awareness field creates space for the expression to move through to completion. Name what their body is doing, including arm movements, posture, tears, and so on.

   You can also do this by naming vocal intonations, tears, or other emotional expressions. Of course, you do not need to do this with every expression. However, when you intuitively sense that certain expressions are communicating something unspoken or are attempting to move stuck energy, naming the expression serves the client's increasing awareness.

2. **Mirror Their Expression:** As you name the client's physical movement, emotional expression, and/or posture, you may also want to mirror it and do the movement, too. For example, if the client placed their hand on their heart, you may bring that into the awareness field by naming it and then placing your hand on your heart.

3. **Name How Their Body Seems:** Being a clear mirror includes being a witness of what the client cannot see. Instead of asking the client what they notice in their body, name how they seem in their body. For example, if you notice tension in their jaw, you can simply name that, and then ask them what they notice there: "It seems like you're holding tension in your jaw. What do you notice there?" This supports the increasing of awareness through direct experience.

4. **Track the Subtle:** When a client is seen for what may seem unperceivable, their awareness increases immensely, and their nervous system feels safe. We will explore subtle energy in later chapters, but for now, the skill is to illuminate the subtle and hold what we're seeing loosely.

   You don't need to be "right" about what you think you're seeing. You simply need to extend yourself in an attempt to see your clients in the deepest, most sacred way. For example, if the client seems to be resisting their emotions, and their throat feels tight, you may say, "It seems like you're capping off your emotion in your throat."

   Alternatively, if a blocked point of energy just seemed to move, you might say, "You seem lighter/softer/etc." Then you may follow that up with, "What are you noticing?" This reinforces that their awareness is the guiding force, and you are a mirror in service of increasing awareness.

5. **Confronting Incongruence:** When a client says something that does not match their physical or energetic expression, or does not match something they have stated prior, it is important to illuminate this incongruence with compassion. In doing so, you support your clients in seeing the way their words are not aligned with their actions, which becomes the entry point for their transformation.

Energetic Witnessing Skills

Energetic witnessing is the skill of giving voice to the more implicit energetic movement. As we listen to our client's words, we also notice their physical movements and posture, as well as their emotional expression. The more they contact their direct experience, the more their energy body (which we will discuss later) starts to reveal its patterns and blocks. As the witness, we can learn to attune to the subtle energy field and honor this insight in collaboration with the client. When we open to the energetic field, we honor the spiritual and transpersonal qualities that are rarely acknowledged in non-therapeutic relationships.

Noticing the subtle ways a client braces against contact, suppresses their emotions, holds their breath, closes in on themselves, leaves themselves, dissociates, and so on supports their shifting levels of consciousness. Their subtle body begins to awaken, and they feel more vital and aligned for having been witnessed.

When we let go of our own thought-based reality, our therapeutic holding is more expansive and attuned than if we assess the client from our mind. We can scan the awareness field and discover stuck or blocked energy that wants to be seen by the client. To do this, we need to be an open vessel. Even the mere suggestion of scanning the field may interrupt total presence and openness, as it may become a thought or inquiry of "How do I do that?"

This ongoing exploration of sensing into the energetic field is a cornerstone of transpersonal counseling. When we are in the practice of giving voice to how the client seems in these moments of arousal or energetic blocks or movement, we are seeing and holding the entirety of the client's experience as sacred.

♦ In bearing witness to the client's subtle energy, we can follow their energy and learn how to direct the movement of their energy in collaboration with them.
   ○ For example, if the client seems self-protected around their heart, we can say, while pointing to the heart center, "It seems like there is a wall of self-protection here." When we give voice to an implicit energetic observation, we own our perception as our own, and we say it with complete curiosity.
   ○ Then, we can see if the client senses that, too. "What do you notice around your heart?" This question highlights that we are completely okay with being wrong, as we are simply attempting to collaborate with the client's deeper experience of themselves.
   ○ If the client notices this, too, then we can guide them into inviting more awareness to their self-protection.
   ○ Inviting them to close their eyes to optimize their interoception, their ability to see their inner landscape, we can invite them to bring more love and compassion to the self-protection.
   ○ As we do this, we find the resonant energy in our system, that part of us that knows what it feels like to be self-protected.
   ○ From this place of deep contact, we may invite them to let themselves feel protected.
   ○ Without trying to change the protection or make it go away, direct the client to bring more awareness, love, and validation to it, meaning to themselves.
   ○ Direct them to take a breath and give it a tone, or ask them, "If the protection had a voice, what would it say?"
   ○ Listen deeply to the subtle energy, and honor what is communicated.

Emotional Validation

Emotional validation is the acknowledgment of a client's feelings and experience as understandable and reasonable. It is a fundamental aspect of the therapeutic container, as it creates a sense of safety and trust. There are two ways that emotional validation can be effective: *Validation from the therapist to the client*, and *validation from the client to themselves*.

Through our presence in the dialogic relationship, our ability to understand and authentically validate the client's experience, we offer confirmation, presence, and inclusion to the client. This is a co-regulating intervention, where empathy creates a sense of contact and safety. When validation comes from the ordinary mind or personality, it may be collusion, where we are agreeing with a false belief held by a client, rather than emotional validation. Similarly, when validation is expressed by focusing on the positive, we may be discounting the client's painful experience and unconsciously encouraging them to bypass their struggle.

Validation honors the client as they are in the fullness of their experience. Direct contact with the therapist through emotional validation offers relational support to the client's process. When a client tries to interpret their feelings, our emotional validation invites them into their phenomenology, where they begin to experience themselves as they are. Instead of cognitively bypassing their emotions, they learn to validate their emotions for themselves. A useful sentence stem in emotional validation from the therapist is, "It makes sense to me that ...." For example, "It makes sense to me that you feel lost." Or, "It makes sense to me that old grief has been ignited from that experience." When our personality is at rest, the offering of validation is a genuine expression of contact rather than an attempt at pleasing the client.

To support their ongoing contact with themselves, inviting the client to validate their own emotional experience creates openings within themselves that are equally regulating and transformative. For example, if the client is sharing about their thoughts of what they *should* do, invite them to take a few breaths of validation to the voice of should, encouraging them to say to themselves, "It makes sense to me that you think I should be different." The moment the client validates the aspect of themselves that resists the actuality of their experience, they become more congruent and begin to regulate their nervous system. Validation has the potential to move them out of story and into their current experience.

Validating their own psychological, emotional, and physical experience interrupts the ways in which a client disrupts contact with themselves and the present moment. This type of validation is not the same as agreeing with the narrative. For example, a client who thinks they're unworthy of love is not to be invited to say, "You are unworthy of love," but rather, to say to themselves, "It makes sense to me that you think you are unworthy ...." When they are able to authentically bring love and compassion to their own distress, they begin to shift levels of awareness. A useful invitation for the client to emotionally self-validate is, "If you're open to this, I want to invite you to turn toward yourself and validate your experience, 'It makes sense to me that you (feel hurt/are angry/long for connection/etc.).'" This supports them in creating openings within themselves for deeper contact with the here and now.

Self-Disclosure

Self-disclosure is an important part of creating a sacred container. Without discernment, self-disclosure can create a murky container filled with projections. With too much attention on the therapist, the therapeutic process becomes thwarted, and the client is often left feeling confused and out of touch with their own sense of knowing. With discernment, contact, and clarity on the *why* of self-disclosure, revealing a personal insight, story, or impact can increase the potency of a container.

Intersubjectivity is the concept of exchanging thoughts and feelings between two people. In a session, this exchange is always occurring on the subliminal or implicit field of awareness. Both the therapist and the client are creating ourselves and making meaning of the exchange in the presence of the other. In this process, the therapist is being affected by the relational interaction as much as the client. Making this exchange conscious allows the "two realities [to] combine to create a third and greater reality" (Mann, 2021).

Intentional self-disclosure is an authentic point of contact between the therapist and the client. When offered in language that owns our experience and perception as ours, revealing our thoughts and feelings can deepen contact while maintaining the sacred boundary. One way to do this is by letting the client know we are impacted and affected by what they shared. For example, we might say, "When I hear you say that, I notice (this feeling/sensation/thought) arise in me. What are you noticing?"

Another way to intentionally present something about ourselves is to share a short and succinct personal story that illuminates the pattern in themselves that they are beginning to see. This is a delicate moment, where our share is in service of the client's learning, and we map their pattern through our own past learning. If we choose to do this, we must explicitly state that we are doing this and ask if they are interested. This supports the clarity of the sacred boundary. For example, "I'd like to share a personal story that might be useful in seeing this pattern more clearly. Are you interested in that?" If it is consensual, it has more potential to truly serve the client.

The key to self-discourse is to offer it sparingly, contactfully, and with great clarity as to what our share is serving.

Use of Questions

Questions have the ability to bring a client out of presence and out of contact with themselves. Alternatively, questions have the ability to bring clients into deeper presence and deeper contact with themselves.

In general, present moment, open-ended questions are the most effective in supporting a client to deepen into presence and contact (Palmer, 2011). Closed or leading questions that are outside of the present moment invite the client to retreat into their mind, seeking narratives to interpret themselves rather than contact themselves. The exception to this rule is closed questions that are present moment and/or clarifying, such as, "Do you feel that right now?"

♦ **Open-ended questions** that are geared toward the present moment invite the client to deepen into themselves. "What" and "how" questions are the most useful in this invitation into presence and awareness. "What are you noticing about yourself right now?" "What do you notice in your body as you share that with me?" "How would you like to use our time together?" "How is that to hear?" "How do you seem to yourself right now?"

  ○ Note: Contact is maintained with the subject *you*, rather than *it*. For example, "How does it feel to say that?" or "What does it feel like to be angry?" are present moment open questions that break contact and encourage depersonalization. Instead, we ask, "How do you feel as you say that?" or "What do you notice as you say that?" or "Tell me more about anger."

♦ **Closed questions** are useful when you're clarifying something, and they are even more useful when they are present moment. For example, if you want to try an experiment (which we will discuss later), you might ask, "Do you want to try something?" This question elicits collaboration and consent, and therefore deepens contact and presence.

♦ **Leading questions are never useful**, and they can be challenging to catch yourself doing in real time. An example of a leading question is, "What would it feel like to forgive them?" or "What would it feel like to bring love to your pain?" Clients cannot answer these questions, as they have not yet had the experience. Instead, you can invite or direct them to do something and then ask them what they notice.

♦ **Questions that bring the client outside of the room** are also only useful for clarifying. Instead of "What do you want to say to your sister?" you can ask "If your sister were here right now, what are the words of your truth?"

Six Intuitive Clairsenses

When our increased awareness is maintained through our communication skills, our personality is at rest, and we have more room to open to the transcendent experience of *intuitive transmissions*. As we hold space from a place of full presence—without merging, projecting, or being overcome by countertransference—everything we experience in the therapeutic container is a reflection of the client. When we are curious about the way our sensations, impulses, and transmissions are a reflection of the client, we gain insight into what is happening for them through subliminal communication. For example, if we suddenly feel afraid, we may be curious why fear is in the therapeutic field. Without assuming it belongs to us, we can honor this as intuitive insight and be curious about the energy of fear within the client.

Learning to develop our intuition and responsiveness, especially in the realm of body awareness and resonance, increases our therapeutic effectiveness (Lobb et al., 2022). Within and outside of the therapy room, we can train our intuition in various ways. Contemplative practices offer us a space to let go of thought-based reality and clear our mind of illusions. Honoring our gut instinct, even when it doesn't make sense to ordinary awareness, increases our connection and trust with our intuitive knowing. Attuning to our body's sensations, spending time in nature, and artistic exploration also elevate our access to intuition. We may even practice asking our intuition for guidance to a particular question. Sitting in silence and opening to the soft answer that sounds unlike ordinary thinking heightens our connection to intuition.

When we practice honoring our intuition throughout our daily lives, we are better equipped to intentionally move from thought-based reality into awareness-based knowing in the therapy room. Gazing up into the Akashic field, which is the interconnecting cosmic field that conserves and conveys the records of past, present, and future (Laszlo, 2007), we can open our consciousness to the consciousness of the universe. We may see nothing, or we may be offered profound wisdom—either way, the simple act of looking makes room for innate spirituality and increased consciousness to be present in the session.

Developing intuition has been found to increase the "quality and depth of the therapist's responsiveness" (Lobb et al., 2022). During sessions, we may be offered a glimpse of intuitive insight. We may hear or see our client's inner young one, or we may see the energetic holding pattern in their pain. We may sense their ancestors, or we may hear the voice of their shadow. We do not contrive the images or insight through interpretation or analysis. These intuitive offerings come forth because we are open to this deep level of presence, awareness, and listening.

To maintain the sacred boundary, we offer our intuitive transmission as a gift. The client gets to decide if they resonate with our gift and want to receive it or if they sense or perceive something else. Intuition is not about being right, as right and wrong are a construct of thought-based reality. It's important that our words reflect the neutrality of our offering. The sentence stem "I think I'm hearing it as …" or "I think I'm seeing this as …" can offer our perspective while communicating that we are not attached to being right about what we are sensing.

Intuition is about opening a dialogue with our clients that makes a deeper level of understanding possible. When we engage in the present moment relationship with our increased awareness, we organically open to our intuitive abilities, as do our clients. There are six intuitive senses, also known as clairsenses:

1. **Clairvoyance:** The ability of clear seeing. Visions, imagery, dreams, witnessing the akashic field, and seeing subtle energy are examples of the clarity we can witness with this sense.
2. **Clairaudience:** The ability of clear hearing. Hearing communication from deceased loved ones, hearing the voice of younger and future versions of our clients, and hearing other people's thoughts are examples of the intuition we can access with this sense.

3. **Clairsentience:** The ability of clear feeling. Sensations in the body, feeling someone's pain, feeling someone's spirit, and having a pang of gut instinct are intuition insights we can gather with this sense.
4. **Claircognizance:** The ability of clear knowing. Knowing about people and events that others wouldn't normally know, such as truths, forewarnings, and so on, are some of the gifts offered with this sense.
5. **Clairalience:** The ability of clear smelling. Odors of a client's past memories and the smell of a deceased loved one can be sensed with this sensitivity.
6. **Clairgustance:** The ability of clear tasting. Tasting something that isn't actually there, like a favorite meal or the memory of a client's experience, can be sensed with this intuitive insight.

Typically, we have one intuitive ability that is easiest for us to access and trust. However, the more we clear our own mind of illusions and open to awareness, the more we begin to access a wider range of intuitive transmissions. The more we honor our intuitive wisdom, the clearer the insight that is offered. The more we ignore our intuition, the quieter it becomes. Intuitive transmission is generative, increasing in intensity and frequency the more we honor its messages.

Learning to use our *experience of the client* as therapeutic insight is a useful transpersonal skill that strengthens intuition in the therapy room. Honoring how we feel as we sit with a client increases our ability to be a clear mirror and gain understanding of the client's inner experience. For example, if you feel unsure that the client is being honest, how can this feeling of *distrust* be made explicit in service of therapeutic transformation? One way to bring *distrust* to the awareness field is to say, "As you're talking, I started sensing a quality of distrust. What do you notice when I say that?" Without narratives as to why the quality of distrust is present, honoring your intuitive senses brings more depth and dimension to the therapeutic process.

When we personalize our experience, we are less likely to share our experience and use it therapeutically. In turn, how we feel stays at the level of the personality and becomes countertransference. However, when we stop personalizing our experience, our intuitive insight becomes a useful therapeutic tool. Thoughts of judgment, the impulse to rescue, feelings of hopelessness, and so on can all be used as intuitive insight into the client's world when we let go of narratives and explicitly welcome that quality into the therapeutic container.

Sometimes, it can be useful to simply make a guess at translating our experience into insight into the client's unspoken experience. By naming what isn't being spoken, we take a therapeutic risk that is either accurate or clarifies what is actually true for the client. Either way, we deepen contact when our full experience is honored in the therapeutic space.

In order to offer our intuition as a gift, we must hold it loosely. The language that we choose is a reflection of this offering being from the purity of our own intuition rather than from our ego. If we think we need to be right, our ego inhibits intuitive offerings. If we trust that our gift is an entry point into something unseen or into a deeper truth of our client, we know that every moment of a session is an opportunity to learn. Language that is useful in this exploration includes, "I'm imagining …" or "I'm hearing that as …" or "I think I'm sensing …" or "I'm curious about …."

Lessons from the Therapy Room

As a teacher, I regularly demo the basic skills of empathetic listening, empathetic witnessing, energetic witnessing, emotional validation, and use of questions. As I weave these skills together with the awareness continuum, students are able to witness the profound experience of being met in the here and now through these offerings. The co-regulation that occurs in a container held by awake awareness can increase a client's access to their inner resources almost instantaneously, allowing them to be more present with themselves and their environment.

In order to be effective at these skills, I needed to be able to shift into awake awareness in therapy sessions (and later in demos). Meeting in the I–Thou, my words land in *the between* dimension, where my offering is greater than what my persona would contribute. Contacting the place within myself where I am not separate from my client, I speak from deep contact within myself. This allows my words to resonate in a way they wouldn't be able to from my ordinary awareness.

As I watch student-therapists practice these skills, I can see when a student is practicing from their ordinary mind or from their most awake, resourced self. From the ordinary mind, a student looks to their practice client as a separate other to figure out. When they reflect, "You feel angry about that," their client retreats up into their mind to figure out if this is true and search for words to explain more accurately. The resonance between thought-based realities seems to be amplified in this interaction, draining the energy of both the therapist and the client.

I recall a moment when a student asked their practice client what they noticed in their body:

> "There's some tension in my heart center," the practice client replied.
> "Does it have a shape?" the therapist asked.
> "Um, it's like a diamond."
> "Is there a color?" the therapist asked.
> "Um, it's … gold?" the practice client guessed.

While the therapist was trying his best at proprioception, he wasn't in contact with his body or his awake awareness. He was looking through the lens of ordinary awareness as he engaged in the I–It relationship, rather than the I–Thou. This turned the questions into a quiz for the client to answer, rather than an invitation to deepen into themselves.

As students build their capacity over the course of their training, they learn to engage in and trust the dialogic relationship. They gain a deeper understanding of the way they disrupt contact with themselves and their environment, and they see the way this impacts their space holding. The difference between sacred space holding and well-executed clinical skills may seem unperceivable, but the impact on the client is the indicator of our capacity to open into awareness and contact clients in *the between*.

Exercise: Sacred Space Holding

In the following exercise, you will practice weaving together the awareness continuum with the skills for sacred space holding. There are four distinct rounds of this exercise, and each round builds on the previous round.

Before you begin, close your eyes and take a few loving breaths. Soften your body and find your seat. Take a few more loving breaths, and open into the field of awareness. Let go of your mind and rest in your infinite Self.

Round 1: Find a practice partner, set the timer for six minutes, and weave together the awareness continuum with reflective listening skills.

For example:

> THERAPIST: "What are you noticing in your body right now?"
> CLIENT: "There's a lot happening … I don't know."
> THERAPIST: "There's a lot here for you in this moment. What do you notice when you say that?"

Round 2: Find a practice partner, set the timer for six minutes, and weave together the awareness continuum, reflective listening, and reflective witnessing skills.

For example:

> THERAPIST: "How is it for you to be here right now?"
> CLIENT: "I'm okay. I'm not sure what to do."
> THERAPIST: "I hear the uncertainty, and you seem to be clenching your jaw. What do you notice there?"

Round 3: Find a practice partner, set the timer for six minutes, and weave together the awareness continuum, reflective listening, reflective witnessing skills, and directing attention.

For example:

> THERAPIST: "What do you notice in your heart?"
> CLIENT: "I feel some tightness there."
> THERAPIST: "I want to invite you to close your eyes and be with the tightness. Let your heart know that you see it, that you see that it's tight."

Round 4: Find a practice partner, set the timer for six minutes, and weave together the awareness continuum, reflective listening, reflective witnessing skills, and directing attention. As you do this, notice how you feel when you sit with the client. Is there something in the field that is unsaid? Use your intuitive insight and see how the client responds.

For example:

> THERAPIST: "What are you noticing now?"
> CLIENT: "My heart is starting to soften."
> THERAPIST: "Your heart is softening. You also seem to be contemplating something. What is pulling the attention of your mind?"
> CLIENT: "I am angry."
> THERAPIST: "Making room for anger. Let me hear from anger."
> CLIENT: "Ugh. I'm so angry that they don't listen to me …."
> THERAPIST: "I keep getting this sense of invisibility. What do you notice when I say that?"

References

Laszlo, E. (2007). *Science and the akashic field: An integral theory of everything.* Inner Traditions; 2nd edition.

Lobb, M., Sciacca, F., Isadoro, S., & Di Nuovo, S. (2022). The therapist's intuition and responsiveness: What makes the difference between expert and in training gestalt psychotherapists. *European Journal Investigating Health Psychology Education, 12*(12), 1842–1851.

Mann, D. (2021). *Gestalt therapy: 100 key points and techniques.* Routledge.

Palmer, K. (2011). Gestalt therapy in psychological practice. *Inquiries Journal, 3*(11), 596–611.

Rosenberg, M. B. (2015). *Nonviolent communication: The language of life* (3rd ed.). Puddle Dancer Press.

Contact

Chapter 6

Contact, the Nervous System, and Spiritual Alignment

Each time we sit with a client, our present moment attention offers them a container to discover the ways they leave present moment awareness and become embroiled in their own thought processes and emotional dysregulation. The meaning they make of themselves and their environment informs our understanding of how they make and break *contact* with the present moment.

Contact is the experience of being in touch with the continual process of our lived experience. It isn't a specific state of being, but rather, the meeting of ourselves and the environment in any given moment (Mann, 2021). When our emerging needs are met by environmental resources, contact is made and our experience is complete, forming a gestalt (Clarkson, 1998). When the environment lacks the resources to adequately meet our emerging needs, we adjust our internal process to create equilibrium. In these moments, contact is disrupted and our need is left unsatisfied, leaving an incomplete gestalt. When the environment is characterized by distressing and disturbing events, our internal adjustment to break contact is influenced by our nervous system response.

When there is a perceived or imagined threat to safety, the neurobiology of our survival mechanism overrides conscious thinking. The energy of our inner resources are preserved to fight or flee, which is called *hyper-arousal*. Hyper-arousal is accompanied with increased heart rate, shallow/quick breathing, tension, vigilance, insomnia, and jitteriness (Porges, 2023). If the perceived threat persists and/or we are unable to regulate our nervous system, ourautonomic nervous system moves into *hypo-arousal*. Hypo-arousal is accompanied by a decreased heart rate, slow/heavy breathing, numbness, emotional paralysis, and sluggishness.

In moments when our internal expereince is overwheleming and we cannot influence the threat in our environment, breaking contact is adaptive. In childhood, when we lack the relational or inner resources to regulate our distressing experience, withdrawing from contact is a wise strategy. When the original threat is no longer present, however, and these strategies persist, the incomplete gestalt influences the way we make meaning. From this place, our patterns of dysregulation remain a baseline in our nervous system, and our strategies to break contact become habits of our personality. Over time, our stress or trauma response cause an impairment in the parietal lobe, which is responsible for access to higher states of consciousness that characterize our innate spiritaulity (Miller, 2023). When traumatic expereinces remain unprocessed, disconnection from higher consciousness persists, causing us to live in a state of disconnection from present moment contact., where wemake meaning-based on the unresolved experiences of ourpast trauma.

DOI: 10.4324/9781003521969-8

When a client arrives to a session in a state of dysregulation, they typically cling to the ways in which they disrupt contact, even though these habits cause them distress. When we are able to hold space from awake awareness, we become the client's *surrogate frontal lobe*, where higher levels of processing takes place. Our presence reminds their limbic system of this same quality within them, inviting them to reconnect with their innate wisdom. By maintaining the seat of compassionate witness, the therapeutic relationship becomes a resource for co-regulation. Through direct contact with us, the client learns to maintain direct contact with themselves. Learning to hold themselves in their dysregulation and discover what is needed, a client can learn to make contact with themselves in a way that is deeply healing. In this process, they learn to expand their capacity to be available for their process and navigate their healing through awareness-based knowing.

Nervous System Regulation

A person's fight or flight response can remain active long after the perceived threat has subsided. In the present moment, a client relives traumas that the brain can't register as belonging to the past (van der Kolk, 2014). The accumulation of unprocessed trauma re-calibrates the brain's survival response, affecting the area of the brain that communicates the embodied sense of being alive.

The role of the amygdala, which is the emotional center of the brain and part of our survival mechanism, is to scan the environment for threats to safety. The four threats to safety that the amygdala senses in the environment are as follows: *Judgment, incongruence, physical threat,* and *the unknown* (Porges, 2023). This environmental scan happens below the level of awareness, and it is increased in clients who have experienced complex trauma.

In general, clients arrive to sessions with an accumulation of unfinished business. The unresolved experiences from the past live within their thought-based reality, their physical bodies, their energetic bodies, and their emotional bodies: When a client is in their fight response, they likely present as indignant or resentful, looping in thought with a high degree of tension in their body and a density to their subtle energy. When a client is in their flight response, they likely present as restless, distracted, anxious, fidgety, trembly, with a tendency to turn way from their experience. When a client is in their freeze response, they likely present as indecisive, full of dread, numb, and stuck. When a client is in their fawn response, they likely present as trying to convince us that they are okay while bypassing their lived experience, and they may seem blank and wide-eyed. When a client is dissasociated, they are likely confused with fuzzy thoughts, feeling detached and ourside of themselves.

Each expression of dysregulation holds a wisdom that communicates the unresolved experience from their past as well as the solution to returning to contact. If we, as a clinician, cannot maintain contact with a client who is dysregulated, we might think that the client needs to be different than they are in order to heal. In these moments, we become a threat to their nervous system. Our desire or impulse to change a client is perceived by the amygdala as judgment, causing our well-meaning intervention to perpetuate dysregulation. Similarly, when we position ourselves in the seat of an expert, a client's amygdala senses the incongruence of our persona and they feel unsafe. When we offer interventions without explicit consent, a client's nervous system can perceive this as a physical threat and they can become dysregulated. There are so many unknowns in therapy, and when we are not in authentic engagement with our clients their amygdala senses that as danger.

Honoring the wisdom of the nervous system, we welcome our clients as they are and listen deeply to what their dysregulation is communicating. Contacting our clients in their experience supports them in contacting themselves. For example, if a client is anxious and talking quickly, we refrain from trying to slow them down or bring them into their body. Instead, we invite them to notice their racing thoughts and bring more awareness into what is present in the here and now. Similarly, a client who is dissociated doesn't need us to try to guide them back into their body. Instead, we can contact them and see them in their disconnection and invite their awareness and soverign will to be the guide of their process. In this process, we are directing the client to come into resonance with their own expereince, which supports them in becoming a safe space for their own healing.

When a client clings to their thought-based reality, they are trying to resolve unfinished buisness while unkowingly perpetuating their dysregulation. Similarly, when we orient toward our clients' narratives, we interrupt their organismic self-regulation. Seeking to understand the client's meaning-making is important for our understanding of what is transpiring within them, as well as for their own clarity. This is a top-down approach to processing, and it is quite useful in creating clarity and openings to contact. Feeling heard and understood is the beginning of co-regulation, and it is one way we contact clients as they are. When we listen carefully to the client's stories, they feel heard and validated as they increase their awareness. It can be useful to invite our clients to close their eyes in order to optimize their interoceptive senses and be the witness of their mind, validating their own experience and contacting themselves as they are.

As we listen to a client's meaning-making, we are paying attention to *what* they are saying. As we track the content of their narratives, it is also important to pay attention to *how* a client seems and *how* they express as they talk. If we begin to interpret or try to figure out *why* a client thinks or feels a certain way, we risk entering into the realm of the I-It and clients will retreat into their mind. Instead, we can invite clients into their present-moment experience by bringing awareness to their body. Sensing into the way their body is holding their experience in the present moment supports access to subtle awareness. This is a *bottom-up* approach to processing, where listening to the body is honored as important for understanding the deeper motivation of the nervous system. As a client comes into direct experience with their bodily sensations, they increase awareness of their inner mind–body process. This invitation teaches clients to honor the wisdom of their nervous system as they process unresolved trauma. As a self-sensing, self-organizing system, this is where they'll discover what it is they need from themselves to find their way through their patterns and back to a state of rest and regulation.

Clients who have symptoms of complex post traumatic stress disorder (C-PTSD), however, may be unable to access their interoceptive sense of their physical body. They may say they *feel nothing* in their body or that *they don't know* what they feel. Desensitizing from one's sensations is an adaptive response to trauma, especially when the threat was persistent and the client had no way of changing their environment (such as in childhood with a volatile caregiver). Having access to their sensations is not a requirement to do this work. In these moments, we have an opportunity to offer some psychoeducation to our clients and guide them in re-sensitizing to their body. This is a sacred opportunity to invite the client to open to their subtle awareness and be in relationship with their desensitization. In this process, we are affirming to the client that we trust thattheir soul knows what it is they need to heal. Honoring the blankness, numbness, or disconnection offers them a pathway on which they can begin to reconnect with their body and discover what it is they need from themselves.

We must not be afraid of dysregulation or see it as a sign of something wrong. Emotional dysregulation is the body's way of communicating its needs. If the client is angry or anxious, we can bring more awareness to the full experience of anger or anxiety, discovering what this emotion needs in this moment. If the client is sad or numb, we can invite them to be with the experience fully or partially, depending on what their window of tolerance can withstand. If the client is trying to convince us and themselves they are okay, we can be with their fawning consciously and illuminate the incongruence, discovering what need lies dormant beneath the people-pleasing. And if the client is dissociated, we can let them know that we see that they left themselves; we can ask them where they went and what they notice in the disconnection. Being with the thoughts, sensations, impulses, and emotions of the experience is the way we listen to the wisdom of dysregulation and discover what is needed to for healing.

Regulation is not better than dysregulation. Regulation is important in that it gives a client rest and resourcing for learning and being present. However, when intense sensations of dysregulation are active, learning to stay connected and engaged with one's self is extremely important for integration. Learning to hold ourselves in our expereince of pain is healing, in and of itself. Regulation is not an outcome-oriented technique. It is the process by which a client expands their capacity to be available for themselves and discover what it is they need from themselves in this moment.

Emotional regulation is the act of being responsive to one's own regulatory needs. This is contrasted by attempting to regulate by suppressing or resisting their experience. By listening deeply to the sensations in their body, clients learn to connect with themselves and be available for their needs. This allows them to return to a parasympathetic state of regulation, where they rediscover a sense of safety and belonging. Clients move from the reactivity of their amygdala into the curiosity, compassion, and creativity of the parietal lobe. This entire process is facilitated by the client's awareness, which is amplified by being seen through our awareness. Our work is to create the space for clients to continue to get more in touch with themselves in each moment and with each sensation, memory, or impulse as it arises.

Developmental Trauma and the Personality

All children have biologically based core needs that they look to their caregiver to fulfill. The needs for connection, attunement, trust, autonomy, and love are essential to a child's physical and emotional well-being (Heller & LaPeirre, 2012). When these needs are met with consistency, a child develops certain capacities to self-regulate and connect with others. When these needs are *not* met with consistency, a child creates adaptive survival strategies in an attempt to find balance in an environment that is not designed for their well-being. This is called *developmental trauma*, where foundational steps of a child's regulatory system and ability to connect with others are disrupted by consistent negligence on the part of caregivers (Heller & Krammer, 2022).

Some of the ways a child adapts to not having their core needs met include the following: Disconnecting from emotions, detaching from the body, disowning their needs, needing to be in control, feeling responsible for others, and having their self-esteem based on appearance (Heller & Krammer, 2022). These strategies were a wise response to an environment not designed for their well-being. However, without the opportunity to develop the capacity to self-regulate and connect with others in a healthy and attuned way, these strategies stay with a person into adulthood and become personality traits. The hyper-arousal of fight and flight, and the hypo-arousal of freeze and fawn, can make their way into personality characteristics in the following ways:

- ♦ **Fight:** Controlling, Explosive, Narcissistic, Bullying, Conflictual, Resentful.
- ♦ **Flight:** Workaholic, Hyper-activity, Anxiety, Panic, Compusivity, Restlessness, Perfectionist.
- ♦ **Freeze:** Confusion, Indecision, Lost, Stuck, Numb, Isolating.
- ♦ **Fawn:** People Pleaser, Codependent, Lack of Identity, Boundaryless, Overwhelmed.

Beneath these characteristics lives the imprint of the dysregulation. In the fight and flight responses, the person's personality perceives a sense of influence or power over the threat, so their strategies are action oriented. In the freeze and fawn responses, a person is unable to influence the threat, so their nervous system moves into hypo-arousal to protect them from experiencing the harm. This is a reflection of perceived power and influence, not gender. Those in power positions perceive the ability to influence relational threats, so they stay in hyper-arousal longer. Those in down-power positions experience the inability to influence relational threats, so they eventually move into hypo-arousal.

When a client begins to come into direct experience with themselves, their subtle awareness allows them to feel the emotional dysregulation beneath their thoughts and behavioral strategies. Understanding the way the personality can express a trauma response offers an entry point for therapeutic transformation. A client who expresses narcissistic personality traits has the opportunity to feel the increased heart rate, tension, and heat of their *fight* response. As they connect with their body, they can sit with the experience of decreased clarity. They have the opportunity to contact their own fear and insecurity. Connecting with themselves, they begin to build the self-trust needed to feel safe and connected to the people in their life.

A client who expresses perfectionistic personality traits has the opportunity to feel the restlessness, fidgety, and shaky feelings of their *flight* response. As they connect with their emotions and their body, they are able to feel the increased heart rate and tension they've been holding. They can sit with their highly distracted mind and reconnect with themselves. As they do, they begin to get in touch with their needs and move through their fears.

A client who is stuck in indecision and loneliness has the opportunity to feel the decreased heart rate, numbness, stiffness, and heaviness of their *freeze*. As they hold their breath, feel lost, or experience a sense of dread, they turn toward themselves and begin to thaw the numbness. Beneath the freeze is often fear and anger, which helps to mobilize out of the freeze response.

A client who expresses a codependent or people-pleasing personality has the opportunity to feel the ways they detached from their body and discount their feelings of sadness of their *fawn* response. When the urge to be responsible for others emerges, they get to be with the experience beneath that impulse. They begin to love themselves in the way they want others to love them. In this work, we prioritize process over pathology, trusting that a client can find their way back to their true nature regardless of their personality habits to break contact. Knowing certain diagnosis is helpful in understanding a client's inner map. With the understanding of our client's unique patterning, we can support them to see that the whole of their inner expereince is greater than the sum of it's parts. Welcoming all aspects of our clients models for them how to expand their capacity to heal their developmental trauma and become present with the here and now.

Trauma and Spirituality

In moments of trauma, a person doesn't have the inner or relational resources to process the event that harmed them. As a person's sense of safety is compromised, it is common for the body to seem like an unsafe space to reside, as this is where they experienced and held the pain. It is also common to feel disconnected from any sense of spirituality and split from their innate wholeness. The more disconnected a client is from their spiritual self and from their body, the more they cling to their mind. Resisting their dysregulation, they create narratives that help them make sense of themselves and their environment.

Being overly loquacious is a common sign of unresolved trauma, indicating that the client has been trying to regulate their nervous system through their mind. However, the nervous system is not connected to our thinking brain, and thus a top-down approach, when leaned on too heavily, can prevent a client from discovering what it is they really need from themselves to repair their system. As the amygdala scans the environment for safety, the parietal lobe closes off to higher levels of awareness, causing the client to move further away from their access to their spiritual Self (Miller, 2023). In these moments, a client looks to the environment to be a source of love, connection, and belonging.

While being in a safe environment is important for healing, looking outside of themselves for the qualities of spirituality that are inherent in their own humanity keeps them giving their power and peace over to others. The manifestation of being disconnected from one's spiritual self is repaired by reconnecting with one's own innate spirituality, and it is not served by trying to get others to provide what they think they are lacking within. When something fundamental to their own spiritual Self, such as a sense of love, connection, and belonging, is sought externally, these thoughts indicate where and how the client can repair their internal sense of spirituality. (More on this in Chapter 7.)

Within the nervous system, there is a nerve, called the *vagus nerve*, which wanders from the brain stem, through the neck, and passes through the chest to the abdomen (Porges,

2023). The vagus nerve helps to modulate stress and trauma responses through breathing, temperature, and heart rate (Porges, 2021). It is the longest and most complex of all the 12 cranial nerves, and it controls bodily responses to stress that do not require conscious thinking, including motor functions in the voice box, diaphragm, and stomach. It is often referred to as the *soul nerve* because of the way it unifies the entire nervous system and in many ways defines what it means to be human (Menakem, 2017).

When the body holds unprocessed stress and trauma, the vagus nerve can become imbalanced, causing physiological and psychological concerns (Porges, 2017). Hypervigilance, increased heart rate, dysregulated breathing patterns, and tension in the body overwhelm the brain and can cause a client to feel confused, lost, and anxious. Over time, if the threat to safety persists, the wisdom of the nervous system turns down the volume on fight–flight. This causes a person to move into a state of decreased heart rate and breathing patterns, causing a client to feel heavy, depressed, and hopeless. In cases of hyper-arousal and hypo-arousal, a person's soul is searching for resolution to unfinished business and a return to their true nature, which is an aware, regulated state of presence.

The nervous system is responsible for almost all areas of a person's functioning, including our sense of well-being and mental health (Porges, 2023). From a regulated state, we experience internal organization, connection, expansion, and aliveness, all aspects of spiritual well-being. From a dysregulated state, we experience a disconnection from life itself and no longer experience the warmth and belonging of our spiritual nature (Miller, 2023).

When a therapist has the capacity to welcome the client as they are and honor the ways in which they adapted, we can make room for their spiritual essence to be the guide of their healing. Honoring that the client's soul knows what it is they need to heal, every expression of dysregulation can become the doorway to find their way back home to themselves. This level of nonviolent space holding acknowledges that some of the medicine the client needs can be found in the way they express their dysregulation.

As we listen to a client's meaning-making and invite them into direct contact with their body, our energetic attunement can track the way the vagus nerve corresponds with energy centers: The *throat, heart,* and *solar plexus chakras*. When a client becomes dysregulated, the emotions that rise to the surface are often experienced as constriction around their throat, a ball in their throat, or a capping off on the upper part of the throat. When a client feels scared or angry, the heart center often feels tight, closed, or constricted. When a client speaks of incongruence, where their will and their authentic truth are not aligned, their solar plexus feels as if there were a rubber band around it.

By attending to these centers with loving awareness, a client is offered space to allow their emotions to move through them, as opposed to holding them in or resisting them. Contacting themselves as they are, they can discover what their nervous system needs from themselves in order to regulate. As their energy begins to move, the client's system may need a tone or a movement or some touch to regulate even more. Where they once resisted or clung to their dysregulation, they begin to open to their experience and allow life to move through them. This allows them to create a new imprint in their nervous system, one where they are connected with their body, their mind is clear, and their innate spirituality flows in alignment with their energy. They return to the fundamental core of their being, and they get to discover how to move in the world from their true nature.

Somatic Intelligence

When a client returns to their spiritual alignment, it is a sacred moment of full embodiment. As they move through their emotional dysregulation, they contact themselves as they are and move through various layers of unfinished business. As they do this, they learn to trust their body's innate wisdom. Learning from the body, they discover what it is they need from themselves to heal and find their way back into full contact.

The body speaks in sensation. Listening to the language of the body offers ourselves and clients a way to access *somatic intelligence*, where we understand information from our physical sensations and use this as a path back to contact (Levine, 1997). With a *top-down* approach to processing, clients express their thoughts and narratives, and we clearly reflect what we're hearing and then invite them to notice the sensations in their body. While some clients are naturally *bottom-up* processors, where they notice the sensations in the body as a means to process sensory information, most need to sort through their thoughts before accessing their somatic intelligence.

Disconnection and disembodiment become a habit. When the body is a source of emotional and physical pain, a client organizes themselves around and away from the pain. Desensitizing from pain becomes the inner motivation for how to manage their experience, which perpetuates the holding patterns of unprocessed emotions. This is known as the *sterile void*, which is a degenerative cycle. The sterile void occurs in a "closed system, characterized by high tension, which leads to insensitivity, which leads to inefficient action, which leads to more insensitivity" (Kaparo, 2012).

The *paradoxical theory of change* reminds us that the more effort a client puts into resisting who they are, the more likely they are to stay the same. The more they fully embody themselves as they are, the more empowered they are to change.

When a client accesses the sensations in their body, they increase awareness of physiological, psychological, and energetic holding patterns. The body and the nervous system have an energetic holding pattern; the mind and thoughts have an energetic holding pattern; and emotional and subtle energy have an energetic holding pattern. The way a trauma response lives in the body must be felt, experienced, and moved through in order for a client to come back to a regulated and aware state. Because of this, a client who is healing trauma may feel worse before they feel better. If they are in a fawning response, they will need to move through their freeze, their flight, and their fight on their way to full presence and regulation.

As a client begins to open to themselves and their body, they unlock their vital force. Eventually, they find themselves in the *fertile void*, which is a generative cycle. The fertile void occurs naturally in "an open system, characterized by minimal tension, which supports sensitivity, which supports efficient and intelligent action, which supports increasing sensitivity and awareness" (Kaparo, 2012).

Somatic intelligence is a pathway for clients to become aware of the way they make contact with themselves and their environment from the sterile void of ordinary awareness. As they fully open to the phenomenology of their experience, they fully embody themselves as they are from subtle awareness. As their awareness increases, they enter into a consciousness beyond the mind, where the fertile void rests in awake awareness.

Co-regulation

Experiencing the co-regulating presence of an attuned therapist offers a client the relational resource they need to find their way through unresolved trauma. When the sensations of the nervous system create great discomfort, it is common for clients to try to control their nervous system by resisting the sensations or turning away from their body. From this state of resistance to their own dysregulation, their experience is amplified, and the dysregulation is perpetuated. This can be experienced as anxiety, racing thoughts, rage, depression, confusion, blankness, and indecision.

When therapists feel discomfort or fear toward a client's dysregulation, we may try to change the client's experience by telling them to take a deep breath or ground. This communicates to the client that their experience isn't welcome here and can actually cause further dysregulation. In these moments, it is possible that the therapist is unaware of how to be available for their own experience, making it hard to be available for the client's.

The sensations associated with dysregulation are the expression of life force energy moving through the body. Rather than working against the client's vital force, we must honor the wisdom of how dysregulation is being expressed. The ways in which a client'senergy has been mistuned by the traumatic experiences they've endured are met with awake awareness, allowing organismic self-regulation to transpire. Pacing a session by moving slowly and making room for each layer of a client's inner experience, we become the relational resource they need to find their way through their distress and back into a regulated, aware state.

Honoring the wisdom of the nervous system, we can teach our clients how to open to themselves as they attend to their inner experience. We do this through our presence and invitations, directing clients into the phenomenology of their sensations from their awake awareness. If the client is in a freeze response, we invite their awake awareness around the experience of numb or empty or desensitized, which supports the thawing of this nervous system response. If the client experiences tension in relationship to the fight or flight response, we support them in wrapping their experience with awake awareness as they discover what they need to mobilize what their nervous system is holding.

The practice of pacing a session through the use of reflective listening, empathetic witnessing, and the awareness continuum supports the client in staying within their window of tolerance, where they have enough activation to repair their nervous system and enough space to think clearly. When clients retreat into their mind and talk "about" themselves or how they "should" be, we contact them in their thought-based reality and let them feel heard. Oftentimes, clients try to regulate their nervous system by creating a narrative that helps them make sense of themselves. As we honor this strategy, we listen to their stories and then gently invite them back into direct experience by asking them what they notice on the level of sensation, even if that sensation is in their head as it relates to their thoughts.

With our attunement and invitations, we are teaching clients how to regulate and be available for themselves, which is the essence of *co-regulation*. Co-regulation is the process by which a client learns to soothe their distressing emotions and sensations through connection with an attuned therapist (Porges, 2023). In the process of co-regulation, clients begin to experience themselves as they actually are, making it possible to experience the world as it is rather than through the state of dysregulation.

Co-regulation creates a space for the client to integrate their past experiences, clear some of their emotional energy, and be loving with themselves. Through direct contact with the therapist, they deepen into contact with themselves. From here, clarity, compassion, and connection to their innate spirituality manifest naturally.

The following are ways to increase awareness as you co-regulate:

- **Bring awareness to thoughts:** Looping in thoughts and clinging to the mind are expressions of a dysregulated nervous system. To break through old stories and discover what is true for themselves, a client must see that they are trying to make sense of their expereince. You can name the narratives with neutral language and invite the client to notice the voice of this narrative. "I want to invite you to close your eyes and notice (that your mind is searching)." This simple invitation invites the client to contact themselves as they are, while also beginning the process of differentiating from the ordinary mind. Instead of trying to get the client to think differently or be more embodied, meet the client where they are. This is the entry point to co-regulation.

- **Bring awareness to their relationship to their mind:** Clients can perpetuate their distress and dysregulation by the way they relate to their thoughts. The two most common distressing ways to relate to the mind are through *clinging* and *resisting*. When a client clings to their thoughts, they identify with their mind and ruminate in their thinking. When a client resists their thoughts, they are identifying with their thoughts, but they judge themselves for having the thoughts and try to make them go away. Simply naming these inner movements increases awareness and supports co-regulation. For example, "It seems like you're resisting this narrative," and then see what the client notices.

- **Bring awareness to the breath:** The breath is the only part of the autonomic nervous system that a client has conscious control over. This makes it imperative for regulation and co-regulation. However, it is important that you meet the breath as it is, without trying to force it to be different. The breath has a wisdom, and you must see the wisdom of the breath to discover what is needed for regulation. Telling a client to breathe deeply when their breath is shallow is not co-regulation—it's an invitation to resist what is occurring within them. By following the breath, you can invite them to notice where the breath naturally wants to go. This supports them in focusing on the breath they are receiving, rather than the places where the breath is restricted. Then, you can invite them to drop the exhale, which makes more room for more breath to enter.

- **Bring awareness to the body:** When a client is in a trauma response, they may not have much access to body awareness. As a co-regulating presence, you can be the witness for them. When offered by an attuned, non-judgmental therapist, naming how a client's body seems to be holding their experience can be extremely co-regulating. As you sit with clients, notice any areas of constriction or openness.

Bring attention to constriction when there seems to be a block of energy ready to move, and bring attention to openness when you want to support them in feeling their own inner resourcing. Always hold your perspective loosely, and always check out the client's experience with them. For example, "It seems like there's tension in your shoulders. What do you notice there?" Once energy has moved, we might say, "Your shoulders seem lighter. What are you noticing?"

♦ **Pause for raw emotions:** Silence is perhaps the most overlooked therapeutic tool. When timed properly, silence can increase awareness, create more space in the container, and support the integration of emotions. Dysregulation is important in the integration of past experiences. As you co-regulate with the client, moments of silence can be a sacred pause where you honor their pain and their ability. It can also be essential for your own breathing and self-regulation. In the silence, you can listen to their consciousness and open to intuition. Learning to stay in the pocket, where silence is spacious but not disconnecting, requires a dedication to the ongoing study of attunement by following the client's energy.

♦ **Make room for discomfort:** As a therapist, if you have not yet learned how to sit with your own discomfort, you may attempt to guide your client away from challenging emotions or experiences. Creating space around discomfort can teach a client how to regulate their nervous system. Supporting or guiding a client to allow their experience to move through them allows a natural catharsis, where old emotional energy can be clarified from their system. Inviting them to open to themselves as they do this offers them space to deepen into contact with themselves.

♦ **Trust the client's inner wisdom:** Perhaps the most co-regulating act you can offer is to trust your client's inner wisdom. When you think you are the expert, the amygdala perceives judgment, and you become a threat to your client's nervous system. When you trust their inner knowing, their ability for self-regulation is honored as a part of their innate intelligence. Everything within a client that is not loved is searching for love. When dysregulation is welcomed by the therapist, the client can make room to welcome the experience with loving awareness. When they can access their inner wisdom in our presence, they can begin to offer their pain the love it's looking for.

Lessons from the Therapy Room

Learning to be in the room with trauma was a capacity I built over many years of practice. As a new clinician, my nervous system would contract and tighten when clients began to feel the emotions associated with their unfinished business. I was afraid of re-traumatizing them, and I didn't trust my ability to support them in navigating their way through their emotional pain. This lack of co-regulation inhibited clients from contacting themselves as they were, as I was unable to contact them there, too.

Committed to my own personal development, I decided to restart my breathwork practice. My mom had been a breathworker, and I had learned this sacred practice at an early age. However, it had been about 15 years since I had last done a breathing session, and the contraction I felt around trauma was an indicator that I was holding my own unresolved trauma.

During my first time back to practicing breathwork, I had a private session where I touched the place within myself where I didn't want to be in my body. My throat closed off to breath, and resistance to my own vitality overshadowed any desire to heal and be alive. A memory of a near death experience flashed into my awareness. I was five months old, and I fell from the top bunk of a bed. The imprint of this experience became the figure, and everything else receded to the background.

As the memory of my infant self was in the forefront of my mind, I kept breathing. I cried, and I kept breathing. My body twisted, and I kept breathing. I felt the pain and terror of almost dying, and I kept breathing. Eventually, I realized that I had been living my life unconsciously orienting toward my pain. I had been clinging to my pain in an attempt to prevent more trauma from occurring, while simultaneously perpetuating my trauma.

With that awareness, I began to relax around my experience. My body was full of the vital energy of my breath, and spaciousness and love surrounded my physical and emotional pain. Spontaneously, my pain began to transmute into healing.

This was a pivotal moment in recognizing the healing power of aware awareness. My relationship to my trauma became loving, compassionate, and spacious. This inner spaciousness I created within myself, in turn, allowed me to create a more spacious therapeutic container. With my expanded capacity to be with my own experience, I expanded my capacity to be with my clients. I learned to stay connected with myself in the presence of trauma, which made it possible for me to stay connected with them when they worked with their trauma. With every part of my being trusting their ability to move through their pain, I also trusted myself to walk through their experience with them. Together, my wisdom interacted with their wisdom, and we could find our way through the inner matrix of trauma together.

Exercises: Finding Safety and Connection

Learning to regulate our own nervous system is necessary in staying awake, aware, and aligned. People often think they are trying to regulate their nervous system when in fact they are attempting to make their dysregulation go away. Resisting our experience is both effortful and dysregulating, as we become a threat to our own nervous system at that point.

There are many ways to regulate our nervous system, and all of them rely on our own capacity to welcome our experience fully. Essentially, we must learn to find safety and connection within ourselves to be available for others. Below is a list of exercises for safety and connection that you can practice alone, with a partner, and with clients.

- Vagus Nerve Massage
  - Begin by placing your fingertips on the top of your head.
  - Make firm contact, not too hard, not too deep. It should feel good.
  - Slide your fingers down the side of your head, around both sides of your ears, down the sides of your neck, toward your sternum and then belly.
  - Use your breath.
  - Repeat as many times as you'd like.
  - If you choose to teach this to a client, consider doing it with them so that you are both regulating and activating your parasympathetic nervous system.
- Stretching the Vagus Nerve
  - After you massage the vagus nerve, elongate the nerve with a gentle twist.
  - Slowly turn toward one side, keeping your hips level.
  - Look over your shoulder, see that no one is there behind you, that you are safe.
  - Slowly come back to center.
  - Then switch.
  - Breathe and repeat.
- Tracking Sensations in the Body
  - Close your eyes to optimize your interoception.
  - Notice a sensation in your body. Even if you feel nothing, nothingness is a quality of the sensation of numbness, so notice that.
  - Refrain from qualifying any sensation as "good" or "bad."
  - Refrain from interpreting why you feel this sensation or what to do about it. Just be with it.
  - Take a few breaths, and then notice the next sensation that arises in your awareness.
  - Stay with your body, and follow the sensations around as they shift.
  - If you choose to guide a client in this process, attune to their breath, body, and subtle energy as you invite them to track their sensations. Pace your invitations to shift to another part of the body in service of co-regulation.
- Pendulating
  - Pendulating is the practice of going back and forth between charged sensations and a neutral or positive one.
  - It is similar to tracking sensations in the body; however, you are pendulating between two specific sensations.
  - Begin by noticing a sensation that feels charged or even painful. Stay with the sensation as you bring more awareness to it.
  - After several moments, look within your body to find an area that is positive or neutral (even if it's your big toe or earlobe). Stay there for several moments.
  - Pendulate mindfully back and forth. Breathe as you continue the practice.
  - If you choose to guide a client in this process, attune to their breath, emotions, body, and subtle energy as you invite them to pendulate. Pace your invitations accordingly.
- Shuttling
  - Shuttling is the practice of moving your awareness from one thought or memory to another.

- ○ For example, you can shuttle between one memory and another, between a memory and the present moment, inner world and outer world, one fantasy or desire and another, or between the dream and now, etc.
  - ○ It is a way of re-owning projected content and strengthening the now. The techniques can be modified to suit what you need; it is a process of experiment.
  - ○ If you choose to guide a client in this process, attune to their breath, body, emotions, and subtle energy as you invite them to track their sensations. Pause in silence before you invite them to shift to the other thought or memory.
- ◆ Proprioception
  - ○ Proprioception is the ability to perceive the location, movement, and action of parts of the body.
  - ○ It's an embodied movement practice where you listen deeply to how your body wants to move and then move from a place of deep contact.
  - ○ It's common to get stuck in rigid patterns of holding the body. In this practice, you will close your eyes, sense into your body, and inquire from a place of contact with yourself about what your body is needing.
  - ○ It can be helpful to do this practice on your hands and knees, keeping the movement going as you breathe and move into areas of stuckness and openness.
  - ○ If you choose to guide a client in this process, invite them to notice where their movement is coming from. As they attune to the shape their body takes, allow your guidance to invite them deeper into the wisdom of the body as they listen deeply to themselves.
- ◆ Orienting
  - ○ Orienting is the practice of mindfully looking around the space you are in and being aware and present with the environment.
  - ○ Very slowly looking around the space, let your eyes land on one item in the room.
  - ○ As you look at that one item, notice at least three qualities of it, three colors or shades, etc.
  - ○ Stay slow and present as you practice this, and then move to another item in the room.
  - ○ This is a wonderful way to invite a client into presence when they are in hyper-arousal or dissociated. As the client orients, ask them to describe three colors they see.
- ◆ Resourcing
  - ○ Resourcing can be useful in creating neural pathways for goodness when the mind is oriented toward trauma, pain, and suffering.
  - ○ The invitation is to remember a time where you felt safe and at peace. It could be on a walk, eating a nourishing meal, sitting in front of the fire, or being with a loved one or caregiver, or something else.
  - ○ As you recall that resource, amplify it by staying there and noticing the body.
  - ○ Using this with a client who is stuck in complex trauma patterns can support them in disrupting the way the mind is orienting to the traumatic events. However, remembering positive experiences may bring up grief. Either way, it is important for clients to access inner resources, such as positive memories, to reconnect with their well-being.

♦ Grounding
  ○ Grounding is the embodied feeling of being connected to the earth.
  ○ The essence of grounding occurs without effort when we can sense into the support of the chair at the lower back or butt, and our feet on the ground.
  ○ Surrendering the exhale, remembering that it takes no effort to be connected to the earth, we can deepen into our groundedness.
  ○ If you are struggling to feel that the earth is there, you can imagine warm, rich soil beneath your feet and move your feet around mindfully until you feel it.
  ○ You may want to take your shoes off and feel the ground solidly supporting you.
  ○ When a client's energy is primarily seated in the upper half of the body, their feet may seem to be floating. This may be a good time to invite them to sense into their sacred connection to the earth and ground.

♦ Attachment to Self
  ○ When sensations in the body feel like they are too big to experience, we may naturally detach from ourselves. The ongoing practice of attaching to Self can support the reconnection and healing in our systems.
  ○ Attaching to Self is where the deepest repair happens within the nervous system, as this is where you can truly discover what you need from yourself and become a secure base for yourself.
  ○ When you are emotionally activated, turn toward yourself and ask, "What do I need from myself right now?" Alternatively, you can turn toward a sensation in your body and ask, "What does this sensation need from me right now?" Attention, love, and compassion guide this self-inquiry on the path of healing.
  ○ When a client seems activated or detached from themselves, you may consider asking them, "What is it that you need from yourself in this moment?" as the invitation to attach to Self. "What does this sensation need from you right now?" is also a gentle invitation that teaches the client how to be available for themselves in moments of dysregulation.

♦ Practicing Your "No"
  ○ A wonderful vagal toning exercise is the practice of saying "no."
  ○ In this practice, you'll need a partner who understands the context of this exercise. Their role will be to ask you to do things for them, and your only response is to say "no" to them. For example, they may ask, "Will you go clean my car?" and your response will be "no." And so on.
  ○ As you practice this, pay attention to your body. Notice where you feel congruence or incongruence in your system.
  ○ To use this with a client, you may want to consider a role play, where you take on the role of a person in the client's life that they have a hard time saying "no" to. In the role play, you will say things that you heard them describe this person saying to them. The client's only response is to practice saying "no."
  ○ When the client practices their "no" in a role play, invite them to slow down and feel their body. If fawning has become part of their personality, they will likely feel a lot of discomfort. Being with this discomfort consciously supports them in vagal toning.
  ○ This can also happen with a pillow, where the client hits the couch with the pillow and yells "No!" However, this type of catharsis is only useful for

someone who is ready to move through the deep in their freeze–fawn trauma response.

- ♦ Finding Resonance
  - ○ Finding resonance is a practice between two or more people where you all close your eyes to optimize your interoception and share three sensations that you notice in your body. As you do this, also describe what you are going to do for this sensation or how you are going to be with the sensation to support yourself in your regulation. Everybody who is present closes their eyes, attunes to the place the speaker is sharing, and does the same thing to their body that the speaker says they are going to do for themselves.
  - ○ For example, "As I close my eyes, I notice that my solar plexus feels as if it's two inches in front of my body. (Takes a long breath.) I am going to place my hand on my solar plexus and take a few breaths. (Silence.) It's still a bit jutted forward so I'm going to move my hand slowly in a circular motion over my solar plexus as I breathe. (Silence.) That's better …. Now, I notice my seat in the chair and I'm a bit lopsided, leaning to the right. (Takes a long breath.) I am going to rock side-to-side slowly and feel into my seat as I breathe. (Silence.) The next thing I notice is my jaw. It's pretty tight, so I am going to bring my fingertips to my jaw and stroke it in a downward motion toward my chin, allowing my jaw to softly open. I'm going to repeat that a few more times because it feels so good." As this person is speaking, the other person or people present will also have their eyes closed and follow along, tending to this same place in their body.
  - ○ After the first person shares three things, the next person goes.
  - ○ Repeat at least twice.
  - ○ Note for when using this practice with clients: As you guide this, eventually share the places in your body where you feel supported to remind the client of their ground.

References

Clarkson, P. (1989). *Gestalt Counselling in Action*. SAGE Publications.

Heller, L., & Krammer, B. (2022). *The practical guide for healing developmental trauma: Using the neuroaffective relational model to address adverse childhood experiences and resolve complex trauma*. North Atlantic Books.

Heller, L., & LaPierre, A. (2012). *Healing developmental trauma: How early trauma affects self-regulation, self-image, and the capacity for relationships*. North Atlantic Books.

Kaparo, R. F. (2012). *Awakening somatic intelligence: The art and practice of embodied mindfulness*. North Atlantic Books.

Levine, P. (1997). *Waking the tiger: Healing trauma*. North Atlantic Books.

Mann, D. (2021). *Gestalt therapy: 100 key points and techniques*. Routledge.

Menakem, R. (2017). *My grandmother's hands: Racialized trauma and the pathway to mending our hearts and bodies.* Central Recovery Press.

Miller, L. (2023). *The awakened brain.* Random House Publishing Group.

Perls, F. (1973). *The gestalt approach and eye witness to therapy* (1st ed.). Science and Behavior Books, Inc.

Porges, S. W. (2017). *The pocket guide to the polyvagal theory: The transformative power of feeling safe.* W.W. Norton & Company.

Porges S. W. (2021). Polyvagal theory: A biobehavioral journey to sociality. *Comprehensive Psychoneuroendocrinology, 7*(1215), 100069.

Porges, S. W. (2023). *Our polyvagal world: How safety and trauma change us.* W. W. Norton & Company.

van der Kolk, B. (2014). *The body keeps the score: Brain, mind, and body in the healing of trauma.* Penguin Books.

Chapter 7

Deepening into Contact

When a client arrives for a session, they are choosing to receive our attention. Whatever external circumstance or internal experience brought them to us, we contact them exactly where they are. If they are sad, we make room for grief. If they are mad, we make room for anger. If they are lost, we make room for disorientation. If they are lonely, we make room for longing. If they are antagonostic with themselves, we make room for self-laothing. If they are dissociated, we make room for detachment. They arrive as they are, we welcome them as they are, and they receive our holding.

Given the quality of our presence, this dynamic, where the clinician is the space holder and the client is receiving our holding, is akin to a healthy caregiver–child relationship. As the receiver, the client's attachment system is offered a reparative experience where they are seen with attunement, empathy, and non-judgment. Although the pain is present now, it is seated in patterns that are attempting to resolve unfinished business. When we shine the light of awareness onto their inner patterns, clients are able to see the internal disruptions they created during moments of unmet needs in the past.

One of the main differences between a parent–child dynamic and a clinician–client dynamic is that it is the parent's job to meet the needs of the child. This is not the case in a clinical setting. It is the therapist's job to hold space for the client, see the client with clarity, and invite the client's own awareness into their internal landscape. Once the client can see themselves more clearly through our reflection, we can guide the client through therapeutic practices where they are able to give themselves what their caregiver was unable to provide. In this way, we teach our clients how to build a secure connection with themselves while being held in the safety of our container.

As the receiver, clients have time and space to move through their internal barriers to connect with their True Self. At the soul level, the client repairs in the deepest way. When the holding is clean and honoring of their sovereignty, we trust that their soul knows what it is they need to heal, and the repair they experience touches every element of who they are. In small and big ways over time, the client reconnects with their innate spirituality and returns to the wholeness of their being. This is a client-led approach to counseling; however, the key is to follow the client's innate wisdom rather than their delusions.

DOI: 10.4324/9781003521969-9

Contact Boundaries

By being present and mindful with the client, we seek to increase awareness rather than intellectual insight. Trusting that the only place to get is more in touch with what's right here, our presence has a meditative quality. This quality of attention is powerful, and it naturally evokes the client's delusions, avoidances, and strategies to disrupt contact (Naranjo, 2004). Internal disruptions to contact that a client creates during moments of unmet needs are known as *contact boundary disturbances*. A contact boundary disturbance is defined as "a habit in which a response (to avoid contact) manifests in the individual's personality even though the original circumstances under which the disturbance may have had adaptive value are not present" (Perls, 1973).

An example of a contact disruption is when a client was punished or threatened with punishment for speaking out as a child. Even though they will not currently be punished for speaking their truth, they still act in a habitual way of avoiding contact by not using their authentic voice.

Contact disruption patterns inhibit a person's ability to perceive the present situation accurately. Clients see the world through the lens of unfinished business, and these lenses create illusions of interpretations that we call narratives. When these narratives make their way into the personality, they affect all areas of life, especially when a client is hyper-identified with their thought-based reality.

Disruption to contact can be seen through the following five psychological constructs and adaptive survival strategies. Because these constructs are part of the human condition, we will explore them through the collective subject *we*:

1. **Deflection:** When we learn to ignore our physical sensations and disconnect from our body, we turn away from contact with ourselves and others. We do this in an effort to block or discharge uncomfortable feelings and thoughts. Disconnected from our body and emotions, we may present superficial contact, putting up an energetic wall, or laughing when we feel uncomfortable.

   Please note that deflection is not the same as not making eye contact. Sometimes not making eye contact is deflecting discomfort. However, other times, it is a cultural sign of respect or a need based on neurodiversity (Figure 7.1).

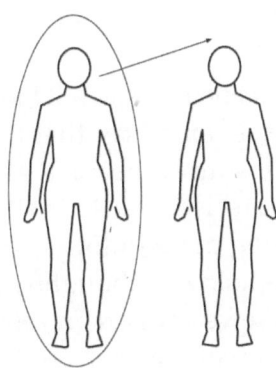

Figure 7.1 Deflection (Kwiker, 2022, p. 112).

2. **Introjections:** When we take on other people's values, ideas, and beliefs without investigating if we truly want them, we internalize ideas that do not belong to us. These introjections become a part of our personality, and we contact ourselves and the environment from beliefs that are not congruent with what we truly value.

    Learned beliefs may also come from the environment and culture, including beliefs about gender, monogamy, money, bodies, racial identities, and privilege. Because these misbeliefs do not resonate with our deepest truth, they cause us distress (Figure 7.2).

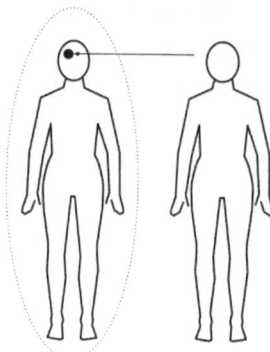

Figure 7.2 Introjection (Kwiker, 2022, p. 107).

3. **Projections:** When we lack the self-awareness of certain unwanted traits or emotions within ourselves and assign these aspects to other people, we are projecting our experience onto others. Projections are an illusion of other people, but they reflect a reality of ourselves and our inner life (Figure 7.3).

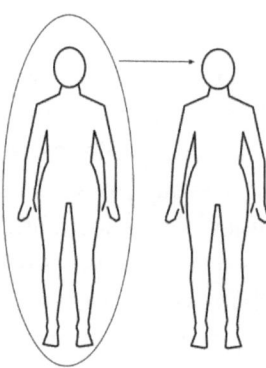

Figure 7.3 Projection (Kwiker, 2022, p. 108).

A projection remains an illusion if we do not look within to see what is occurring in our lived experience. This is not to say that the world around us is not doing the thing we are observing; it simply means that when we are projecting, we are denying something within ourselves. As Perls (1973) states, "We live in a house of mirrors, thinking we're looking out windows."

4. **Retroflection:** When we withhold our thoughts, emotions, and actions from others, and instead put them on ourselves, we are in retroflection. For example, if in childhood we experienced our caregivers as untrustworthy, it was not safe for us to tell them that we needed to have more integrity. Because we did not have space to

express this need, we put it on ourselves to have the highest integrity. For this to be retroflection, we would do this to the extent that the mind criticizes ourselves in an effort to have the most integrity. Retroflection often sounds like the voice of an inner critic (Figure 7.4).

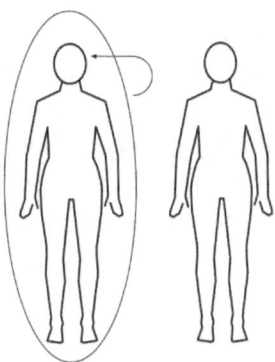

Figure 7.4 Retroflection (Kwiker, 2022, p. 111).

5. **Confluence:** When we do not have a sense of self and do not know where we end and others begin, we are confluent with our environment. Merging with others causes a lack of differentiation, which in turn causes us to take on other people's thoughts and feelings. From a state of confluence, it is common to unconsciously think, "If other people are okay, I am okay." When in a state of perpetual confluence, a person is susceptible to gaslighting, where they feel confusion about reality and allow others to dictate reality at a cost to themselves.

    Please note that confluence is not the same as a collectivist culture taking care of one another. To be truly confluent, we need to feel distressed by a lack of sense of self (Figure 7.5).

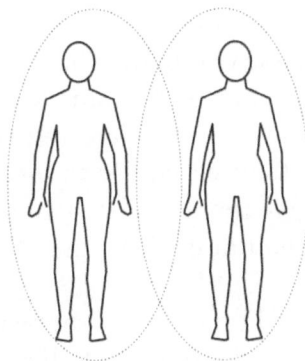

Figure 7.5 Confluence (Kwiker, 2022, p. 110).

The psychological constructs that cause a client to disrupt contact with themselves and the present moment become the therapeutic entry point. This is known as the *figure-ground theory*, where the client's therapeutic content (figure) offers insight into how they make sense of themselves, while the undifferentiated context of their life (ground) is the foundation of the figure (Mann, 2021).

Understanding contact boundary disturbances informs the therapeutic process. However, it is not necessary or even recommended to name contact boundary disturbances to clients. When we maintain process over pathology, we can utilize this insight in service of contacting a client at the place in which they disrupt contact, and this becomes a guide for them to come back into contact and presence.

When a client is fully present and in contact, these disruptions to contact have positive expressions: Deflection is a way to ease tension and find safety; introjection is the ability to take in other people's ideas and perspectives; projection is the place where intuitive seeing resides; retroflection is self-accountability; and confluence is the transpersonal experience of honoring our interconnectedness. When they embody presence, awareness, and clarity of mind, these gifts of the human mind emerge as healthy expressions of their healing.

Homeostasis and Homeorhesis

It is part of the human condition to disrupt contact with ourselves and the environment, especially when we feel unsafe. We do this in an attempt to find inner and outer balance in a system that is imbalanced. When this attempt to create stability in our environment (via disrupting contact) becomes rigid ways of being, this is known as *homeostasis*.

Homeostasis literally means to "to maintain a stable internal environment between interdependent elements," (Merriam-Webster, 2023). When a client creates patterns of disrupting contact, they are adapting to a painful experience of unmet needs from the environment. When they continue to use these patterns even though the original circumstances are no longer present, their homeostasis becomes the rigid pattern that is attempting to prevent the pain from continuing.

It is common for clients to be unable to identify the ways their needs weren't met, because accepting their circumstances was part of the survival strategy. Children, being newly embodied, look to their caregivers to be a safe landing space and to offer them a sense of belonging. In many ways, they see their caregiver as the all-knowing, all-giving Creator of Life. When their caregiver fails to give them a consistent sense of safety and belonging, they unconsciously rationalize that it is their fault. This gives them a sense of power in a situation where they feel powerless.

By continuing to hold patterns of homeostasis, the way a person engages in the present moment is seated in the past. Ultimately, the adult client unconsciously looks to others to fill the role of the all-loving Creator of Life. Patterns that are rooted in the unconscious belief that the belonging and safety they long for comes from others create a false center. To disrupt these patterns is to disrupt homeostasis. We disrupt homeostasis not only through our contact with the client but also by externalizing these inner constructs in the therapy room through experiments (more on this later).

Once we begin to discover a client's rigid patterns that were created to *create equilibriam*, we can support them in discovering *homeorhesis*, which is where the health of their vital force thrives in a steady flow of continual development and adaptation. As opposed to a closed system that ineffectively keeps a client in a state of stress, a client opens to themselves and learns to listen to their body as they deepen into contact. In a state of homeorhesis, a client effectively regulates their nervous system and moves fluidly with life.

Energetic Boundaries

Contact happens at the boundary point in relationship to one's environment. Boundaries are often thought of as barriers or walls, but in truth, they are the place where relationship contact happens. When we, as clinicians, practice embodying our flexible energetic boundaries, we are able to meet clients at their contact boundary.

When a clinician is accustomed to feeling and sensing their environment with great acuity, their boundaries may be open or confluent. Merging with our environment is not contact, for it is a lack of boundary. This makes for a murky therapeutic relationship, where it becomes challenging to decipher where we end and the client begins.

Similarly, when a clinician stays guarded or inauthentic, cautious to let themselves be affected by their environment, their boundaries may be too rigid. Keeping the environment out is not contactful, for it becomes a barrier to connection. This makes for a very clinical container, where the therapist engages with the client as a separate other.

When our energetic boundaries are toned and healthy, our nervous system is regulated, and we are in full contact with ourselves. Knowing how we feel as a separate being, we know what we want and what we value. From this place, we are clear about where our energy ends and where our client's energy begins.

In Figure 7.6, we can see three different types of energetic boundary systems: open, closed, and flexible.

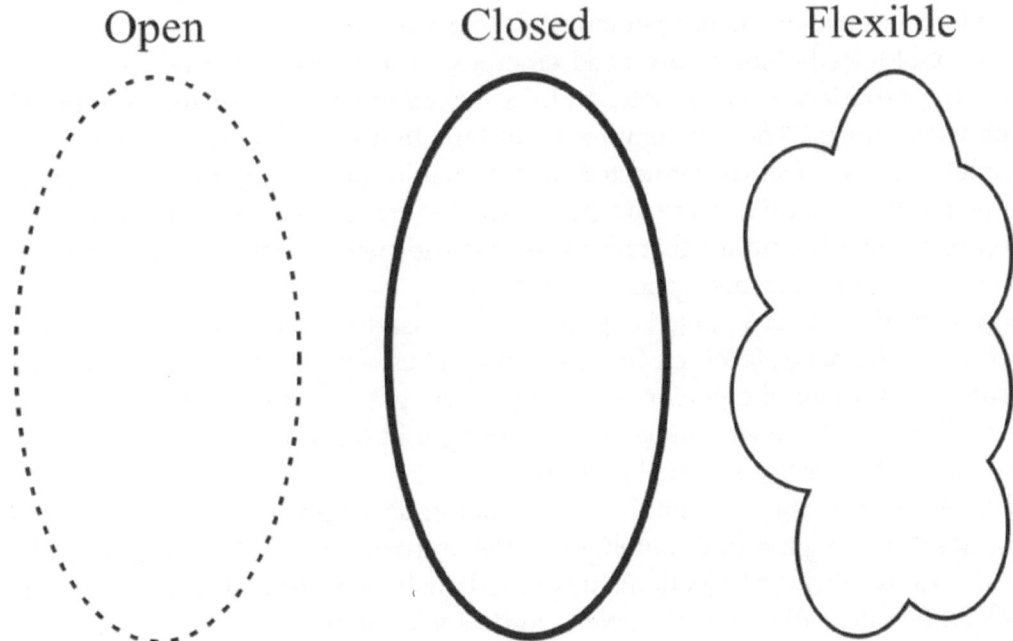

Open   Closed   Flexible

Figure 7.6 Energetic Boundaries (Kwiker, 2022, p. 200).

When we have flexible, healthy boundaries, we hold no therapeutic agenda. An agenda is a predetermined outcome. When we think we know what the client needs, our agenda disrupts contact. From a healthy energetic boundary, we may want something for the client. For example, we may want to support a client in clearing an introjection or working with their confluence. However, if we hold this to be the agenda for a session, we override a client's sovereign will. Asking a client what they want, and then sharing what we want for them, allows us to navigate the therapeutic interventions consciously and collaboratively.

When we are able to stay connected to ourselves throughout a session, our energy flows up the midline of our body, and our boundaries are clear and clean. When we trust our client's connection with their Source of energy, healing, and wisdom, we contact them at the boundary point. This is essential in preventing burnout: Remembering that we have our own Source of energy, and that the client has theirs, instead of giving our energy away, we journey with our clients as they find their way back into alignment with their own Source of energy.

Cycle of Disrupted Contact

The *Cycle of Disrupted Contact* illustrates the way incomplete experiences cause us to create habits that disrupt contact with our environment. The cycle, as depicted in Figure 7.7, shows a series of inner experiences that arise when the environment fails to adequately meet our emerging biologically based core need, such as a need for connection, autonomy, attunement, trust, and love (Heller & LaPierre, 2012). Combining concepts from interpersonal neurobiology with the *Gestalt Cycle of Formation and Destruction* (Clarkson, 1989), this cycle clarifies the meaning-making that occurs through interactions with environment, as well as the way unresolved experiences influence personality structures.

When a biologically based core need emerges, and the environment adequately meets that need, the experience is complete, and we feel connected, regulated, autonomous, and in contact with others. When the environment fails to meet our core needs, the experience is incomplete, and we feel disconnected, dysregulated, burdened, and out of contact with others. The patterns that we create during times of incomplete experiences contribute to the formation of contact boundary disturbances and the subsequent misbeliefs and strategies that are at the root of those disruptions to contact.

The cycle begins when a person experiences a sensation that indicates a need for contact (Clarkson & Caviccia, 2013). When that person reaches out for social or biological support, and the need is not met, the person adapts by turning away from their own emotions and sensations (deflection). Deflection becomes a strategy to disrupt contact, and disconnecting from themselves becomes a habitual pattern.

In this experience, they perceive others as being unaccepting of their desires or needs, and they adapt by denying their autonomy. This, in turn, causes them to personalize other people's ideas and values (introjection). Introjected misbeliefs become part of their personality patterns as they internalize other people's words and actions.

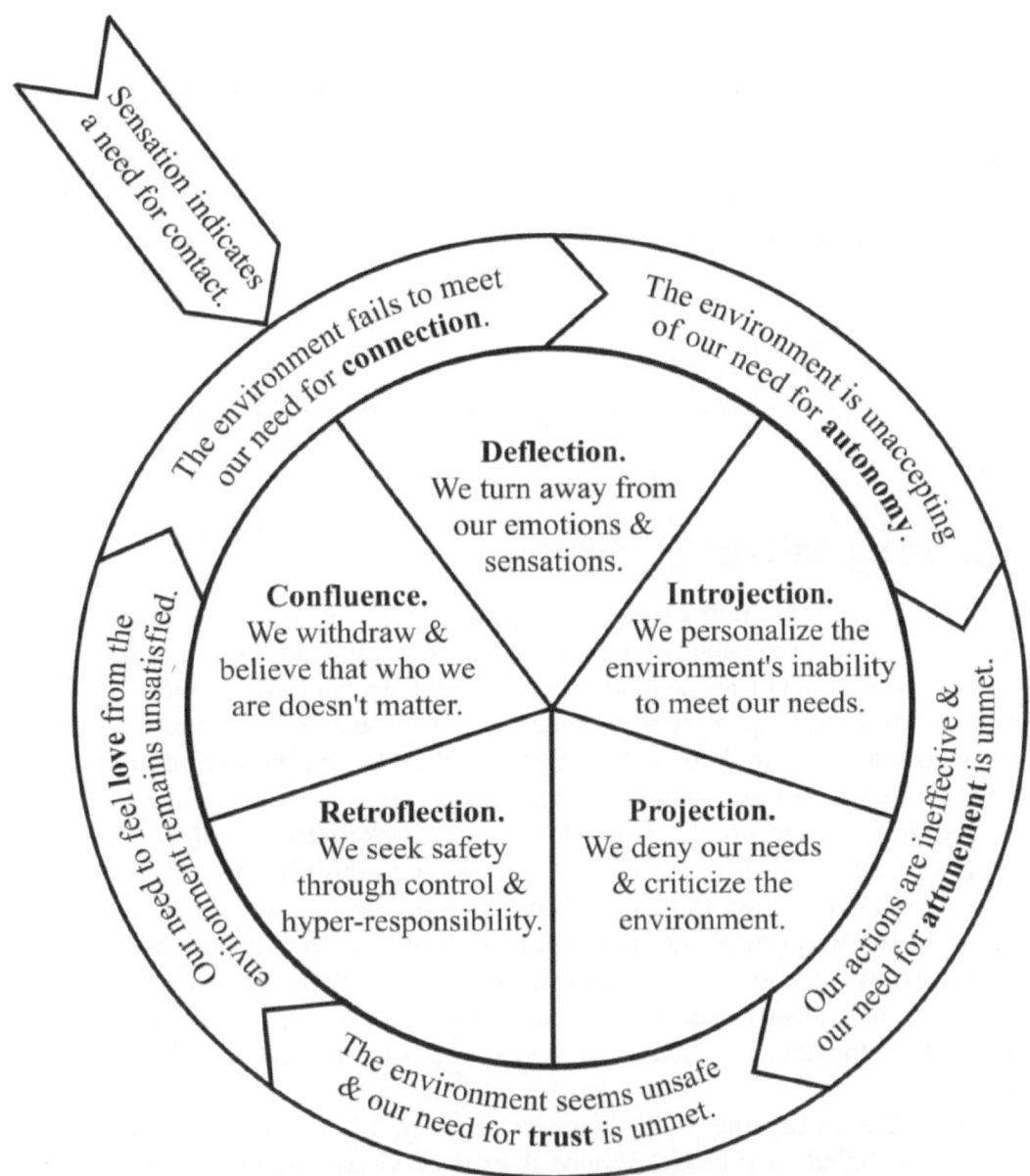

Figure 7.7 Cycle of Disrupted Contact.

Since their actions to get their needs met are ineffective, they adapt by believing their needs do not matter. They disconnect from their needs and assign their inner experience to others (projection). Projecting their experience onto others, they misplace their needs and instead, criticize the environment as a personality strategy.

Because the environment seems unsafe, they seek safety and control by withholding self-expression. Believing they cannot trust others, they adapt by putting onto themselves what they needed from others (retroflection). Retroflecting becomes a personality trait where self-criticism and hyper-responsibility replace self-expression.

When the need for contact is left unsatisfied, the person withdraws and believes that who they truly are doesn't matter (confluence). Confluent boundaries become a strategy to find safety by merging with others. As a personality trait, they prioritize others as more important than themselves.

One incomplete experience in childhood where our needs are unmet by the environment can make its way into our personality and influence our thoughts, emotions, behaviors, and sense of well-being. Each of the five contact boundary disturbances has this one experience embedded within it.

Contacting What's Here

As we learn the client's patterns of disrupted contact, we begin to see the thoughts that pull them out of presence and into the habits of the ordinary mind. This nonviolent approach to therapy honors the wisdom of how the client adapted during distressing experiences in the past and utilizes the mistuned energy or vitality embedded in those adaptive patterns. The medicine the client is seeking actually lives within the thoughts that cause them distress. Instead of interpreting or analyzing those distressing thoughts or behaviors, we listen to the intelligence that exists within them and use that to guide the client back to the core of their being.

For example, if a client is frustrated that the people in their life are incompetent, we can begin to listen to the mistuned and blocked energy that dwells in this unresolved frustration. As we listen to the wisdom of the frustration, we can discover what is at the root of this experience and how it guides the way a client disrupts contact. By honoring the client's innate spirituality and energy body, their patterns of distress and disruption to contact become the doorway to where the light of awake awareness enters. Organically, they find their way back into alignment.

Much of a client's healing takes place when they are able to give themselves what the environment failed to provide. Where they needed connection, we support them in connecting to themselves. Where they needed autonomy, we support them in honoring their will and sovereignty. Where they needed attunement, we support them in learning to attune to themselves. Where they needed safety and trust, we support them in building self-trust by being a safe place for themselves. And where they needed love, we invite them to open into loving awareness within themselves. Whatever is present, we make room for the experience and invite the client to be available for themselves in the way they needed others to be available for them.

While there are likely many unresolved experiences and correlating contact boundary disturbances, we begin with the most predominant or accessible construct. Pictured in Figure 7.8, we see an image of a person who gets pulled off center from their alignment by the way they relate to their unfinished business. This is the very thread we use to support them in finding their way back home to themselves.

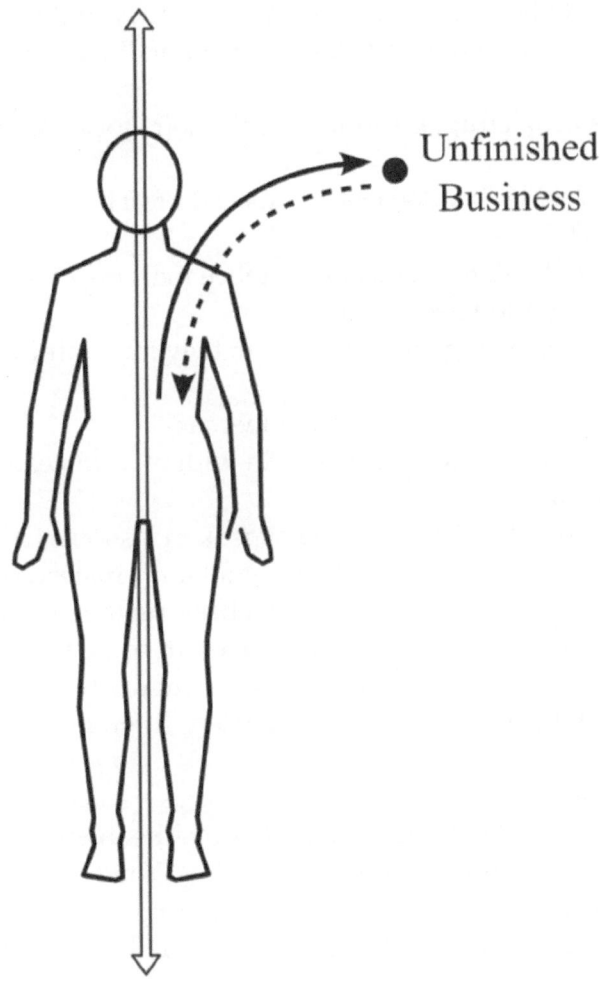

Figure 7.8 Deepening into Contact.

Language Patterns and Contact

A person's words express the energy where their awareness is seated. When their awareness is intertwined with what is unresolved, there are certain language patterns that express these contact disruptions (Bottome, 1976). Contact boundary disruption can be heard through the way a client denies personal responsibility, depersonalizes, objectifies, or resists what is. Learning to hear the way a client's language is shaped by their emotions can serve as an access point to deepening contact.

Common language patterns spoken by clients include the following:

♦ When a client is in **confluence**, they will likely use *you* or *we* instead of *I*.
  ○ Example: "*You* feel like *you* just can't go on," instead of "I feel like I just can't go on."
  ○ Example: "We all want to feel heard," instead of "I really want to be heard."

- ◆ When a client is **deflecting** or **depersonalizing**, they will likely use *it* instead of *I*.
  - ◦ Example: "*It* feels good to say that," instead of "*I* feel good having expressed that."
- ◆ When a client is **projecting**, they may couch their stories about others in feeling language.
  - ◦ Example: "*I feel like they* don't care," instead of "They seem not to care, and I feel sad about that."
  - ◦ Example: "*It feels like they* don't even notice me," instead of "I have a story they don't notice me, and I feel resentful."
- ◆ When a client is expressing an **introjection**, they may minimize themselves and their experience.
  - ◦ Example: "I'm *just* sad," instead of "I feel sad."
  - ◦ Example: "I *only* want them to check in with me," instead of "I want them to express their care for me."
- ◆ When a client is **retroflecting**, they may speak in a shouldism.
  - ◦ Example: "I *should* be further along than I am," instead of "I want to keep learning" or "I wish my caregivers had been further along before they had me."
  - ◦ Example: "I wish I was (different than I am in some way)," instead of "Now that I see the way that I am with more clarity, I am ready to transform (this aspect of myself)" or "I wish my caregivers had been different than they were when they had me."
- ◆ When a client **objectifies** others, *it* can be used as a substitute for *them* or *you*.
  - ◦ Example: "I don't like *it*," instead of "I don't like them/you."
  - ◦ Example: "It seems unfair," instead of "They/You seem unjust."
- ◆ When a client exaggerates, they may be expressing a **cognitive distortion**.
  - ◦ Example: "They *never* listen to me," instead of "When they seem not to listen to me, I feel enraged."
  - ◦ Example: "It's *always* a struggle," instead of "Sometimes, being in relationship with them feels like a struggle."
- ◆ When a client is not in touch with their autonomy, agency, or choice, their words express a **helplessness**.
  - ◦ Example: "I *have* to go to their house and help them," instead of "I want to/I get to/I'm choosing to go to their house to help them."
- ◆ When a client **gives their power away** to others, they may speak in language that points to victimhood.
  - ◦ Example: "I want them to (be different in some way)," instead of "I am ready to show up differently in this dynamic."
  - ◦ Example: "I don't know why this keeps happening to me," instead of "Given this repetitive situation, I want to find my contribution to the dynamic."
  - ◦ Example: "They're so full of themselves," instead of "I want to know my own importance and value."
- ◆ When a client is beginning to **dissociate**, when their nervous system is outside of the window of tolerance, or when they have a history of gaslighting, their mind may go blank.
- ◆ Example: "It's so confusing" or "I'm so confused" are indicators to slow down and bring awareness to confusion.

Our clients' words inform our understanding of their deeper emotional and psychological state of being. As we are listening, we have an opportunity to increase awareness through our reflections and invitations. Here are some ways to work with these language patterns:

♦ **Confluence:** When a client uses the subject *you* instead of *I*, you can simply reflect what they said in the language of responsibility: "You feel like you're going to explode with anger."

♦ **Deflection:** When they use the word *it* instead of *I*, you can reflect it in the language of responsibility: "You feel tense."

♦ **Depersonalization:** When they use the word *it* instead of *I*, you may ask them to repeat what they just said in the language of responsibility. Ask them what they notice what they do this. These moments can support deepening of contact and increasing awareness: "Say that with the word I … I feel …."

♦ **Projection:** When they are expressing a projection, use your reflection to unblend their feeling from their narrative: "It sounds like you have a story that they forgot about you. How is that for you?" or "When they seem this way, how is that for you?"

♦ **Introjection:** When a client minimizes themselves, reflect their experience in a contactful way: "You're sad right now."

♦ **Retroflection:** When a client resists how they are, ask them what they want: "I heard you say you should go to the gym. Do you want to go to the gym?"

♦ **Cognitive Distortions:** When they speak in absolutes and exaggerations, reflect their words back to them with more space around them: "It *seems* like they never ..." or "It *seems* like they always …."

♦ **Helplessness and Powerlessness:** When a client expresses a sense of victimhood, listen for the unmet need beneath their words: "I'm hearing it as … I really want to know that that I matter." Or "I'm hearing this as, 'I want to feel powerful.'" Alternatively, when they say they *have* to do something, ask them if they want to.

♦ **Dissociation:** When clients are confused, pause and make room for confusion: "I want to invite you to stay with confusion. Let yourself feel confused."

The interplay between a client's language patterns, emotions, and unfinished business offers a therapeutic entry point that can be the precipice of deep transformation. Working with language helps us to keep the therapeutic container clean of unconscious energetic patterns. It is also important that we use language of responsibility in our lives to hold the energetic quality of self-responsibility and ownership over our experience.

Lessons from the Therapy Room

In my own life, my cycle of disrupted contact began when I was four years old. At this time, my father came into my room and told me he would be living in a different house.

As he walked out the door, my mom was in the other room crying hysterically and my sister ran up to me and told me it was my fault. Because I didn't have the inner or relational resources needed to process the experience, I disconnected from my sensations (deflection). I internalized the misbelief that people leave because I am inherently unlovable (introjection). I disconnected from my needs and viewed other people as not enough for me (projection). I worked to have high levels of attunement and competence because I did not feel safe to ask my caregivers to be more attuned and competent (retroflection). And my sense of self was intertwined with making sure that others were okay (confluence). While these patterns were a wise attempt at creating balance in an unwell system, when they became rigid characteristics of my personality they were an outdated effort to create homeostasis.

Learning to stay in contact with myself in the presence of others was some of the deepest work I have done on my personal growth journey. In both my personal and professional life, my inability to fully contact the environment was a reflection of my own unfinished business. My contact boundary disturbances were inhibiting my ability to be fully present with my clients, and I was eager to discover how to find a new and truer way to be in the world.

In 2017, I found my way to a community center where they taught and practiced a relational meditation called *authentic relating*. Authentic relating was created from a combination of integral theory, gestalt theory and a group practice called T-group, which was created at Stanford University as a way to confront implicit biases and internalized racism with humanity and authenticity. There are various authentic relating games and practices, all of which offer a training ground to discover contact and self-responsibility.

One of the practices that I trained in was called *circling*. In many ways, circling is a gestalt group practice led by anyone who is interested in being in contact in the present moment. The guidelines for circling included the following: You needed a group of three or more people who were willing to commit to 30–45 min of being present with one person (the circlee). This was a relational meditation practice, the circlee was the focus of the meditation, and their only role was to be themselves and share what they wanted. The role of the other participants was to be curious about the circlee and *get their world*. As the participants stayed present with the circlee, they also needed to *welcome everything* about the circlee, *share impact*, and *own their experience*. These principles mitigate projections and cultivate contact.

When I first started the practice of circling, I would tremble in my trauma response, afraid that others would chastise me or discard me. Over time, as I shared my authentic truth with strangers, I began to stay in contact with myself and contact the world at the contact boundary. Moving through deflections, illuminating introjections, noticing projections, being witnessed in retroflections, and undoing patterns of confluence, I found a way to transmute my contact boundary disturbances and be fully present with life.

With each contact boundary disturbance I transmuted, my capacity to hold space for clients expanded as well. Once I was no longer disrupting contact, I was able to see the way my clients disrupted contact with clarity. I was able to stay present and in contact through every moment of a session, and I was able to fully access my intuitive wisdom as the guide for my interventions.

Exercise: Cultivating Healthy Boundaries

Set an energetic boundary:

1. With your eyes closed, use your hands to feel into your full energetic space.
2. Breathe into that space and push out energetically from the core of your being. This may look like using your hands to push outward, creating a bubble of sorts.
3. Take up all of the energetic space that is yours.
4. Then, tap your sternum with the fingertips of one hand as you put the other hand in front of you as a stop sign.
5. As you do this, visualize a person in your life who needs boundaries. See them as if they are sitting on the other side of your boundary.
6. Envision this person in their own bubble.
7. Tell that person, "I am here, and you are there."
8. Notice how you feel as you contact them at the boundary.

References

Bottome, P. (1976). A gestalt way of using language. In J. Downing (Ed.), *Gestalt awareness: Papers from the San Francisco Gestalt institute* (pp. 104–111). Harper.

Clarkson, P. (1989). *Gestalt counselling in action.* Sage Publications.

Clarkson, P., & Caviccia, S. (2013). *Gestalt counselling in action.* Sage Publications.

Heller, L., & LaPierre, A. (2012). *Healing developmental trauma: How early trauma affects self-regulation, self-image, and the capacity for relationship.* North Atlantic Books.

Kwiker, H. (2022). *Align: Living and loving from the true self.* Mantra Books.

Mann, D. (2021). *Gestalt therapy: 100 key points and techniques.* Routledge.

Merriam-Webster.com Dictionary. (2023). *Hemostasis.* Retrieved January 21, 2023. https://www.merriam-webster.com/dictionary/homeostasis#:~:text=ho%C2%B7%E2%80%8Bme o%C2%B7%E2%80%8Bsta,an%20organism%2C%20population%2C%20or%20group.

Naranjo, C. (2004). *Gestalt therapy: The attitude and practice of an atheoretical experientialism.* Crown House Pub Ltd.

Perls, F. (1973). *The Gestalt approach and eye witness to therapy* (1st ed.). Science and Behavior Books, Inc.

Chapter 8

Resonance and Polarity

Energetic resonance and polarity occur between therapist and client, as well as within the client themselves. Resonance between the therapist and the client manifests when the vibrational quality of the client is matched by the therapist (Wadsworth, 2022). Resonating with the client's lived experience, our limbic system communicates to theirs full trust in their inner wisdom (Vetere, 2023). This degree of trust invites the client to also trust their process, inviting them to deepen into the actuality of their experience. When they fully accept themselves as they are, they begin to find inner resonance, where they resonate with their lived experience without resisting or clinging.

When a therapist is not finding resonance with their client, we are holding an energetic polarity, or a quality of opposing energy (Wermer, 2014). One way a therapist holds a polarity is by positioning ourselves as an expert. If we are the expert while the client is lost or suffering, we unknowingly prevent the client from discovering their own inner expertise. Another way a therapist becomes a polarizing force in the clinical space is by placing our attention on a different construct than a client's current experience (Young, 2017). For example, if a client says they want to do more to heal their patterns, and we focus on how much inner work the client has done (without first reflecting what they've said), we are holding a polarity. Similarly, if a client says they are not feeling resentment anymore, and we ask them to express resentment, we are holding a polarity.

If we are holding the polarity, we unknowingly occupy the inner opposing energy that exists within the client, inhibiting a client's opportunity to do their own work. When enough resonance is cultivated between the therapist and client, confronting their shadow can support them in contacting their inner polarity. By gently illuminating or reflecting the blind spot we observe in their inner map, they can begin to integrate their shadow. The safety that is cultivated with resonance makes confronting a client's blind spot more palatable (Sheldrake, 2009).

Energetic Resonance

Resonance is a synchronous vibration that matches the energetic quality of another vibration (Sheldrake, 2009). When we come into resonance with a client, we are energetically meeting

DOI: 10.4324/9781003521969-10

them where they are without merging with their experience. The tendency to become absorbed in confluence is common in highly sensitive clinicians. Learning to use our felt sense experience *of* the client therapeutically allows our heightened sensitivities to become our super power. Remembering that we are, in fact, a separate human being from our client is what paradoxically allows us to utilize the transpersonal realm of *oneness* to navigate the session with our experience *of* the client as our guide.

The skills of holding a sacred container (Chapter 5) support cultivating resonance between the therapist and the client. When we reflect the client's words back to them, we are expressing a form of resonance, where the vibration of our words matches the vibrational quality of the client's words. Empathetic and energetic witnessing is also a form of resonance, where we see the client for their whole experience as they are in the moment and meet them in their energetic vibration. Subtle attunement is a deep form of resonance, where we feel the client's experience in our body without leaving contact with ourselves.

When a client is in the midst of a deeply distressing emotional state, our resonance communicates empathic harmony and strengthens their self-regulatory processes (Fiskum, 2019). Beyond our words and our witness, finding resonance within our felt sense accesses our intuitive wisdom through our physical sensations. When we are in the resonant field of awareness, the energy of our felt sense resonates with a client's energy. Embodied resonance allows our system to become akin to a tuning fork, where our presence illuminates the vibrational quality of the client's energetic holding patterns (Mckusik, 2021). The awareness cultivated in this process makes it more possible for the client to work with their energy blocks.

Tuning forks measure the vibration of sounds and energy while matching the frequency in order to return the energy to its natural quality (Beaulieu, 2010). To match the frequency of the client's sensations, we simply need to be aware of any new physical sensations we feel as we sit with our client. We then ask the client what they notice in this specific part of their body. Alternatively, if the client states that they feel a sensation in their body, we bring our awareness to that same part of our body. Staying with the felt sense of resonance allows us to enter into the phenomenology of the client and discover what the energy needs.

Having our own inner reference point to what a client expresses, our empathetic capacity supports co-regulation that is beyond words or interpretation. When our resonance amplifies stuck energy in the client, they begin to see and experience their holding patterns with more acuity. Instead of fighting their energy or judging their energy, we invite them to be with themselves in a way that cultivates inner resonance. If judgment is the strongest energy, we invite them to resonate with *judgment*. If they think they should be different, we invite them to resonate with *should*. Whatever is present is met with the quality of sameness, which allows them to meet themselves as they are and find their way back to the natural frequency of their energetic expression.

Ways to find resonance:

♦ Reflect your clients' words. Their words said back to them encapsulate a quality of sameness that allows you to find resonance.
♦ Reflect your clients' emotions. Their emotional expression named and reflected back to them creates a sense of resonance.

♦ Feel the quality of their experience in an area of your body. This is not transference when you know it belongs to the client and use it therapeutically. It becomes valuable intuitive information when you explore the resonant field.

♦ Feel into your somatic experience in the client's presence. When you have a baseline of how you feel before a session, finding resonance with the client's experience becomes easier.

♦ Be curious about how your felt sense might intuitively resonate with the client's felt sense. With your inner eye, bring attention to your own somatic sensations, and then inquire about this physical space in your client's body.

♦ Ask the client what they notice in a part of their body that you feel in your body. Even if they feel nothing, your resonance has brought that quality into awareness. This may be useful at a later point in the session.

♦ Tell the client how they seem. Your attuned eye offers deep resonance.

♦ Validate without colluding. Validation can be useful in finding resonance. "It makes sense to me …."

♦ Breathe up the midline of your body. The more regulated you are, the more you become aware of inner constrictions and blocks within the client.

Ways to invite the client into resonance:

♦ Invite the client to validate their own experience. For example, if a client is feeling angry, you might have them close their eyes and turn toward their anger, inviting them to say to anger, "It makes sense to me that you're angry."

♦ Invite the client to wrap their inner experience with love. For example, if a client is feeling tense, you may invite them to turn toward the tension and breathe the breath of love around tension. Validation can again prove useful here if you invite them to say to themselves, "It makes sense to me that you're tense."

♦ Invite the client to express their emotion: Speak from the voice of anger, give fear a tone, and so on.

♦ Invite the client to give their inner tension patterns a voice. For example, if their heart is tight, ask them to express the phenomenology of the tension: "If your heart had a voice, what would it say?"

♦ Invite the client to repeat their words and notice what they feel in their body.

♦ Invite the client to exaggerate or repeat a movement they made or a shape their body took and notice what they feel in their body.

A word of caution for the new therapist: When a client has a personality disorder, finding resonance with them is only useful if you have clear and solid boundaries. Personality disorders have a strength to them that can induce the therapist and create a cloudy container if energetic boundaries are not set. Focus on using your reflective statements to find resonance and give your client back their own stories and narratives. In this way, their work remains with them and does not stick to your energy.

Identifying a Polarity

A polarity is made up of two contradictory aspects that oppose one another (Stone, 1999). When we hold an opposing vibrational quality from the client, we unconsciously manifest within the therapeutic relationship what is theirs to feel internally. The energy of the session can easily become stuck when the therapist and the client are in contradictory positions. Unknowingly, we become a threat to the client's amygdala when we attempt to change their current experience. Subliminally communicating to the client that they should be different than they are, we inhibit the container from being a sacred place for them to explore their inner world.

When the client cannot see beyond their distress, the therapist acts as the client's surrogate frontal lobe, where we support the client in expanding their vantage point beyond the limits of their current state. To remain calming and reassuring without holding the polarity of the session requires that we find resonance with the client before we present the alternative or confront the polarity. Our resonance can sing to the client's amygdala, allowing their limbic system to regulate in our welcoming presence. To find resonance with the client while also seeing their wholeness, trusting their process, and looking at the larger landscape of their map requires that we stay embodied and regulated as we hold space from awake awareness.

Once we find enough resonance to create safety in the container, we will organically begin to see the shadow or the polarity within the client. When we've maintained a clear witness and reflection, the client's internal polarity emerges naturally. The polarity is typically comprised of the predominant pattern of their ordinary awareness, meaning the aspect of the mind they are hyper-identified with, and their shadow experience that they resist. This is called the top-dog/under-dog dynamic (Perls, 1973). The top-dog is where societal "shoulds" live, and the under-dog is where their resistance to societal demands lives. One aspect becomes the mask, while the other aspect dwells in the shadow.

Inner polarities are two opposing qualities of the personality that seem to be at odds with one another. *When a polarity exists, both aspects of it block the person's energy and cause distress.* A polarity creates inner tension and distorts vital force from flowing in alignment with their true nature. A polarity is not something "negative" opposing something "healthy." For example, if a client wants to create healthier habits, but they procrastinate, this is not a polarity. Procrastination blocks energy, and t needs to be opposing some other energy within the client to be a polarity: Perhaps, procrastination opposed by perfectionism.

Learning to identify a polarity requires that we are curious about the essence of what is beneath a client's presenting problem. If a client arrives to a session saying that want to experience joy in their life, we must not assume that we know what *joy* means to the client. Finding resonance with the client, we first reflect and invite them to share more: "You have a longing for joy. Tell me more."

As the client speaks, we can listen for the inner constructs that prevent them from experiencing what they want, known as their primary strategy and their shadow strategy. Continuing to find resonance with the client, we reflect what we think we're learning about their primary strategy: "As I'm listening to you, it occurs to me that you have a lot of attention on other people. What do you notice when I say that?" This reflection is an observation of their primary strategy, not their specific words.

If the client agrees with this observation, they will likely go on to talk about how they track other people and take on the caretaker role in their relationships. Staying present with them, we can invite them to deepen into their experience by asking, "What do you notice in your body as you share that with me?" By looking within, a client has the opportunity to discover what is beneath this predominant pattern of their personality and to discover their shadow strategy.

If the client notices tension or frustration in their body, we can invite that frustration to have a voice. "Tell me more about frustration." In this invitation, we are following the client's energy and making room for the full range of their experience. They might say, "I want someone to care about me!" Because this desire lives beneath their primary strategy, it lives in their shadow.

Inviting the client to find resonance with themselves, we can invite them to feel the longing for others to care about them in their body. "Closing your eyes, let yourself feel the longing for care." In this moment, the client is beginning to offer themselves what it is they long for from others as they care for themselves.

Now that enough resonance has been cultivated, we can name the polarity: "I think I'm seeing this as, 'I take care of everyone else, and I want to be taken care of by others.' What do you notice when I reflect that?" It's important that we explicitly name what polarity we think we're seeing and check it out with the client. Collaborating with the client to identify their polarity honors their agency and ensures that the work we do moving forward is aligned with the truth of their experience.

Steps to identify a polarity:

♦ Whatever the client brings to the session is the presenting symptom.
♦ As you find resonance with the client through your reflections and invitations, begin to look for their primary strategy.
♦ Continue to find resonance by reflecting what you're learning about their presenting symptom and primary strategy. Invite the client to deepen into contact with themselves with the awareness continuum.
♦ Begin to identify the shadow strategy that lives in the client's blind spot.
♦ Reflect your observation of the way their shadow is polarized against their primary strategy.
♦ Check in with the client to see if this observation fits for them. Collaborate with them to find the right language for the essence of the polarity.
♦ Once you and the client have explicitly identified the polarity, you can set up an experiment (which is outlined in Chapter 11).
♦ Through your experiment, you will support the client in unblending the polarity. This process is necessary for increasing awareness and mobilizing energy that keeps the client in habitual patterns of distress. When each aspect of the polarity is explored separately from the other, the client is able to differentiate from their main strategy and illuminate their shadow strategy.
♦ Towards the completion of the experiment, clients will naturally arrive to a place of integration, self-compassion, and self-responsibility (Figure 8.1).

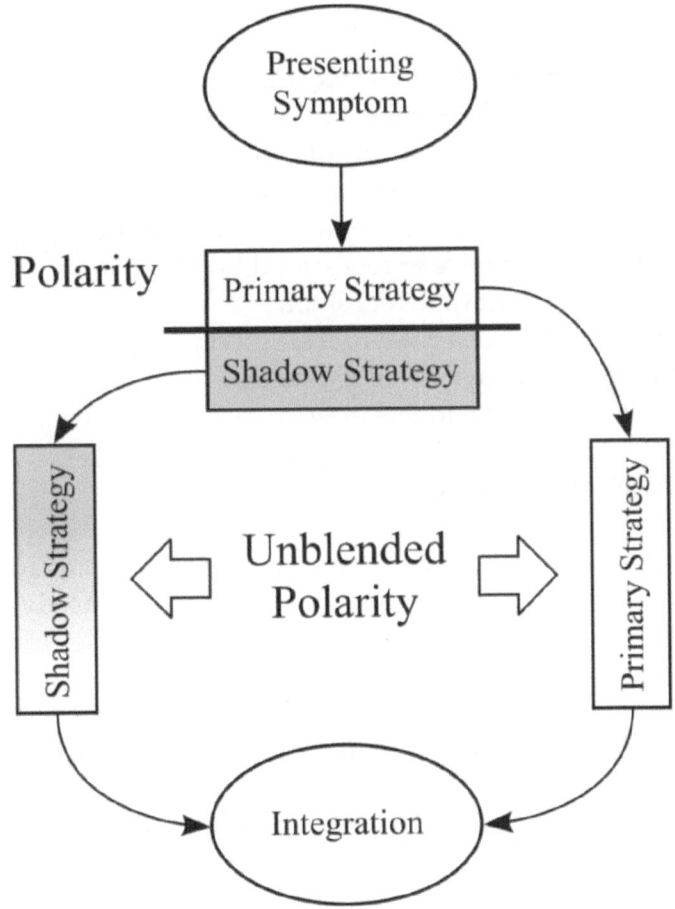

Figure 8.1 Polarity

Common Polarities

The presenting issue the client arrives to a session with is often an expression of one aspect of their inner polarity. Wrestling between their main strategy, known as the top-dog, and their shadow strategy, known as the under-dog, causes the client various levels of distress (Perls, 1973). The main strategy is typically the pattern developed to find belonging and safety during their development. The shadow strategy is typically the desire, fear, or shame the client resists.

Below is a list of common polarities clients present with. In this list, polarities are offered as internal patterns or other-referenced patterns. The language used in these lists is to signify the internal way a client relates to their primary strategy and shadow strategy, and it is not indicative of the actual words the client will say:

Internal patterns of polarities:

- ♦ I cling to perfectionism so I don't feel worthless.
- ♦ I cling to perfectionism so I don't feel out-of-control.
- ♦ I cling to busyness so I don't feel insignificant.
- ♦ I cling to loneliness so I don't have to feel vulnerable.
- ♦ I cling to self-righteousness so I don't have to feel out-of-control.
- ♦ I cling to control so I don't have to feel scared/helpless.
- ♦ I cling to blame so I don't have to feel shame.
- ♦ I cling to resentment so I don't have to feel responsible.
- ♦ I cling to deceit so I don't have to feel powerless.
- ♦ I cling to logic so I don't have to feel inferior.

Other-referenced patterns of polarities:

- ♦ I want others to see me as perfect so they don't see me as trashy.
- ♦ I want others to see me as perfect so they don't think I'm needy.
- ♦ I want others to see me as selfless so they don't think I'm self-centered.
- ♦ I want others to see me as proficient so they don't think I'm ignorant.
- ♦ I want others to see me as accommodating so they don't think I'm demanding.
- ♦ I want others to see me as strong so they don't think I'm weak.
- ♦ I want others to see me as accomplished so they don't think I'm a failure.
- ♦ I want others to see me as special so they don't think I'm boring.
- ♦ I want others to see me as loyal so they don't think I'm disposable.
- ♦ I want others to see me as virtuous so they don't think I'm wicked.

In an individual client, the polarity is internal, between their primary strategies and their shadow strategies. When working with couples, the polarity is reflected in each person, where each embodies what the other has disowned. For example, one person in the couple is self-sacrificing, and the other is self-centered. Another example is where one person is spontaneous and spends a lot of money, and the other person is more deliberate and frugal. The work of each person is to integrate what their partner is reflecting in order to create more balance within themselves. For example, when the person who is self-sacrificing owns their desires, and the person who is self-centered develops care and empathy, each person is more balanced, and the relationship is healthier.

When working with groups, the general group field typically resonates with all group members, but one person holds the dissonance and embodies the polarity. For example, the group may all agree that they like meditation, and one person holds the energy of dislike for mindfulness practices. At first, the group field may feel off balance, but once all people have space to voice the truth of their experience, integration and fullness begin to permeate the field.

Polarities are also mirrored on the level of society, where society is polarized between values and beliefs in an attempt at creating a narrative that gives a person a sense of certainty (Klein, 2020). Creating a bridge of understanding, where humanity is honored with curiosity, we begin to create a more balanced society where people are no longer vilifying one another.

Finding Resonance with the Polarity

Finding resonance with the client is important in making room for their inner polarity to emerge. As we do this, we also invite the client to find resonance within themselves through practices of self-compassion. Once the polarity is identified, the client must find resonance with both aspects of the polarity in order to increase awareness.

When we have a shared understanding of a polarity with our client, creating distance between the two opposing aspects can support increasing awareness. Invite the client to place one aspect of their polarity in a different chair, or invite them to imagine one aspect is sitting in front of them (these experiments will be explored in detail in Chapter 11). When they have the space to unblend the polarities, they are better able to find resonance with each aspect of the opposing energy.

If the client's current polarity is "I want others to see me as selfless so they don't think I'm self-centered," we would collaborate with them to distill this polarity down to its essence. The essence of this polarity would likely be a main strategy of *self-sacrifice* polarized against a shadow strategy of *disowned needs*. In this case, we would invite the client to speak from self-sacrifice. After they have expressed the voice of self-sacrifice, we would invite them to notice how they feel in their body. Attuning to the energetic holding pattern of self-sacrifice, they can begin to find resonance with this main strategy. Welcoming the wisdom of this strategy, they become a safe space for themselves to explore their shadow strategy.

Once the client has found enough resonance and increased awareness of their main strategy, we may invite them to move into the seat of their shadow strategy. Expressing the sentiment of voice of disowned needs, we can invite the client to experience the felt sense of this shadow strategy. Finding resonance with the shadow illuminates it with the light of awareness, and the energetic holding pattern of the polarity begins to soften. The inner tension releases in the presence of the client's ability to resonate with their opposing energy.

Lessons from the Therapy Room

I've learned over the years that in order to identify a client's polarity, I need complete trust in the wisdom of the way they are organized internally. There are times when a polarity appears, and it is clear and neat. In these sessions, the unblending process is quite easy, as the polarity is easily defined. Other times, a polarity is all tangled up inside, and it is messy and chaotic. In these sessions, unblending the polarity requires skillful presence and deep curiosity in order to define it accurately.

I was once working with a client whose inner polarity was quite chaotic, and she was fatigued by her tendency to get tangled up in her own inner world. She was quite intelligent and could see other people's patterns very easily. When it came to herself, however, she circled in the same inner and outer patterns, feeling tremendous shame for not making the changes she wanted for herself.

One day, this client arrived expressing her shame for being in the same position as she had been the week prior. As I listened, I began to map out her polarity as being stuck between her *low self-esteem* and her *accountability*. While this polarity seemed clear to me, internally, these two constructs were so intertwined that their seemingly conflicting messages came out in everything she said.

"Are you open to trying something?" I asked.

"Yes," she said, looking tired and defeated.

"I want to offer that we do a two-chair exercise with the voice of low self-esteem and the voice of accountability. Are you up for that?" This client had done several two-chair experiments in the past, so she had an understanding of what I was suggesting.

"Okay."

"In the chair to your right, let's put the voice of low self-esteem, and the chair that you're in will be the voice of accountability. Take a moment in this seat and let yourself feel the energy of accountability. What do you notice?"

"I'll just say what's here … it's like, I don't want to be accountable because no one is. Where are all of the adults? If I hold everyone accountable, I will be alone."

"What do you notice in your body as you say that? 'I don't want to be accountable … where are all of the adults? I'll be alone if I'm accountable.'" I could see here that low self-esteem was merged with accountability, so I invited the client into her present moment experience to support deepening contact, which helps the unblending process.

"I'm so lonely."

"Close your eyes and let yourself feel alone." She started to cry, and I supported her in moving through the grief. "Accountable, sitting across from you is low self-esteem … the voice of 'I'm not worthy of good people,' what would you say to them about why you're here?" To further support the unblending process, I had her look at the other seat and speak directly to it. Visually seeing the separateness can be helpful to clients in this process.

"Ugh … I am trying to protect you. I don't want anyone to see you. If I can get them to be accountable, we'll get love."

After she voiced this, I invited her into her body with the awareness continuum. We stayed here for several moments to continue to unblend the polarities before I invited her to switch seats.

"Notice how you feel now that you're in the seat of low self-esteem. Accountability over there said that they are trying to protect you. They don't want anyone to see you. They want you to feel loved. What do you notice?" I reframed what the other seat said in order to highlight that these are two different constructs holding two different consciousnesses.

"I feel so much shame. It's like I'm trash … the lowest of the low."

"And how does accountability look to you from here?"

"They are so rigid and judgmental. They are zealous in their righteousness and push people away. Their standards are too high, and no one will ever meet them." This was new information about accountability. The client started to cry, and I supported her in allowing the grief to move through her.

"Is there anything you want to say to accountability?"

"Yes, what you're doing isn't working. We are alone, and I don't know if anyone loves us."

I invited the client to switch seats. When she was in the seat of accountability, I reflected what low self-esteem had just said. Over the course of the experiment, she touched the place beneath accountability to long for love. She also touched the place within low self-esteem that has dignity. Low self-esteem held their ground with accountability, and accountability heard her in an authentically loving way.

"Now, I'd like to invite you to take a third seat," I offered, "the seat of your wise, awakened Self." The client moved to the third seat. "From here, I invite you to look at these two aspects of yourself. Is there anything you want to say to them?"

She started crying and placed her hands on her heart, "I want to welcome them home."

"I invite you to take a few breaths and welcome them back into your heart. In the form they are in now, with dignity and softness …."

After the experiment was complete, the client could see that accountability was actually the younger strategy, holding everyone to high standards. She could also see that low self-esteem, when in balance, held energy that was quite powerful and full of dignity. She needed the dignity from the part of her that she had been disowning in order to balance out the voice of accountability. And, she needed the humility of the balanced accountability in order to bring greater balance to low self-esteem. By taking the time to unblend these aspects of her inner polarity, she was able to discover for herself, by herself, what was keeping her at an impasse.

Exercise: Naming Your Polarity

This next activity invites you to explore your own polarity to support you in being able to identify them in your client. To practice identifying polarities, use these two sentence stems. You can use them alone, with another person, or in a group. These sentence stems are powerful invitations that get to the essence of polarities quickly. Sharing yours and hearing others' helps to normalize this inner experience, which eliminates shame and supports healing.

"I cling to _____, so I don't feel_____."

"I want you to see me as _____, so you don't think I'm_____."

Notice how you feel as you identify your polarities. Stay connected to your body as you discover the way your patterns pull you off center from the core of your being.

References

Beaulieu, J. (2010). *Human tuning: Sound healing with tuning forks.* Lightning Source Inc.

Fiskum, C. (2019). Psychotherapy beyond all the words: Dyadic expansion, vagal regulation, and biofeedback in psychotherapy. *Journal of Psychotherapy Integration, 29*(4), 412–425.

Klein, E. (2020). *Why We're Polarized*. Avid Reader Press/Simon & Schuster; Illustrated edition.

McKusik, E. D. (2021). *Tuning the human biofield: Healing with vibrational sound therapy* (2nd ed.). Healing Arts Press.

Perls, F. (1973). *The Gestalt approach and eye witness to therapy* (1st ed.). Science and Behavior Books, Inc.

Sheldrake, R. (2009). *Morphic resonance: The nature of formative causation* (4th ed.). Park Street Press.

Stone, R. (1999). *Polarity therapy: The complete collected works* (Vol. 1). Book Publishing Company.

Vetere, A. (2023). Coming full circle with the neuroscience: Using new theory to re-understand therapy. In T. Grover, U. Axberg, & S. M. Myra (Eds.), *New* horizons *in* systemic practice *with adults* (pp. 163178). Palgrave Macmillan.

Wadsworth, C. F. (2022). *The fundamentals of resonance repatterning*. Resonance Publishing.

Wermer, H. W. (2014). *Mysticism, physics, polarity and mother earth: A physicist's report on his mystical experiences*. Books on Demand.

Young, P. (2017). *Polarity therapy: Where energy meets structure and function*. Masterworks International.

Chapter 9

Mapping the Client's Inner World

Clients are multidimensional beings with a vast and unique inner world. When they become stuck in the habits and conditioning of their ordinary mind, they can feel confined to an incomplete experience of themselves. As therapists, we can support a client's transformation by exploring the territory of their inner world and illuminating conditioned thoughts and habits. This helps them to differentiate from the ordinary mind and bring awareness to alternative options so they can find their way home to their true nature. When discovering new territories, it can be helpful to create maps of the landscape being explored. As therapists exploring the inner world of our clients, we can also become map makers as we explore our client's territory.

A client's map is a symbolic representation of their familiar and often limited way of relating to themselves and their environment. As map makers, we learn the unique territory of our clients and make mental notes of important landmarks. We must be careful not to mistake the map for the territory, lest we confuse "the semantics of a term with what it represents" (Korzybski, 1933). Each inner construct that causes a client distress becomes a marker on our understanding of their inner map. If our map making is accurate, its structure is similar to the client's inner territory, which accounts for its usefulness in navigating their configuration of distress patterns.

When a client orients to a map that was created during times of stress and unmet needs, they restrict themselves to a portion of territory that no longer serves them. Familiar patterns of thinking and behaving keep them circling these outdated territories as they try to find their way into new experiences of being alive. Where a client feels limited by their inner map, we are able to see the larger landscape in which their strategies exist. The pathways and trails that pull a client further away from who they are become the very trails we follow as we help them find their way back to themselves. Acceptance and awe of the client's multidimensional wholeness remains the guiding principle throughout this process, for we aim to see not only patterns of distress, but the brilliance and beauty of their infinite Self as well (Clarkson & Caviccia, 2013).

We are not learning a framework and placing it onto the client, for the map maker never tries to move the territory around. Instead of using the map to get from point A to point B, we learn the way each landmark on the map is interconnected with the whole of the territory. We do not try to move the mountain to where the lake is or the lake to the flatlands. We simply want to get a lay of the land and understand the territory as it exists. If the map expands and shifts, it does so because the elements support this transformation. A client's awake awareness (sunshine), emotions (rain), breath (wind), and sovereign will (fire) transmute their map into an environment designed for their well-being.

DOI: 10.4324/9781003521969-11

The unique patterning or configuration that comprises their map forms a gestalt, where together each pin or landmark is greater than the sum of its parts (Kaffka, 1935). Considering that each landmark relates to all of the other landmarks, we uphold the primary values of the I–Thou relationship, where our authentic engagement in the healing process honors the client's wholeness (Mann, 2021). Each time we sit with a client, maintaining a beginner's mind, or *shoshin*, allows us to let go of our preconceptions and maintain an openness in our awareness (Suzuki, 1973). This attitude contains both doubt and possibility, where we have the ability to always see our clients as fresh and new. Although we know their map from previous sessions, we also see their developing sense of self, where their map is a dynamic and ever evolving understanding of their inner territory.

Understanding Maps and Landmarks

Mapping a client's inner world is a creative process that supports them in developing self-awareness (Cole, 2022). It is a process by which we learn the various ways a client relates to themselves and the environment, as well as the birthplace of any disruption to contact. Any idea or impulse that pulls a client out of alignment with the core of their being becomes a marker on the map, along with any resources or innate wisdom that is present. In order to see a client's map clearly, we must be able to understand the lenses that they view their inner and outer worlds through. Identifying their belief systems embedded in their narratives, behavior, emotions, somatic experience, and spiritual aspects of their life allows us to understand the various landmarks that comprise their unique map.

While we learn a client's unique inner territory, we listen for the deeper essence of what underlies each landmark, consistently holding their perspective in mind when working with them (Zinker, 1978). Each landmark holds insight into the client's perception of stuckness, as well as their liberation. Unfinished business, distorted energy, disturbances to contact, blind spots, and deep wisdom are embedded in the pins on their map. We welcome both the "dark and regressive aspects of being human and also of our innate striving towards health, happiness and self-actualization" (Clarkson & Caviccia, 2013).

A client instinctively perceives distressing thoughts as being in the foreground, while everything else recedes to the background. This is known as the *figure-ground principle*, where the objects of the foreground are the *figure*, and the undifferentiated background is the *ground* (Mann, 2021). The figure is the landmark that we work with, and the ground is the terrain in which we explore the multidimensional wholeness of their being. The characteristics that make up the figure become a therapeutic entry point on our journey of navigating their inner world.

Once we've gathered enough information about the specific characteristics of certain landmarks, we can practice *zooming out* to see the larger territory, or ground, in which these landmarks exist. With our expansive and compassionate vantage point, we can guide the client through the terrain of their map. Where the client feels stuck at the foot of a mountain, seeing only what is in front of them, we can see the larger picture and the various trails available to them.

Discovering the Map

Mapping typically begins with gaining understanding of the habits and patterns of a client's ordinary mind. This is where we can discover the delusions or misbeliefs that cause the client distress. Themes of perfectionism, indecision, resentment, or blame may emerge. Misbeliefs around being unlovable, broken, or cursed might be present. Ideas that evoke patterns of self-betrayal, self-loathing, or lack of self-trust might be found here. We might discover cognitive distortions, where the client *always* feels left out or thinks they *never* get what they want.

Each idea is a marker that identifies an element of the client's inner landscape that they use to navigate the world. We learn if they are seeing themselves and the environment through the lens of unfinished business. We learn if they tend to be antagonistic with themselves. We have the opportunity to listen for the ways they personalize the way other people treat them. And, we gain understanding of the ways they might unconsciously believe they are fundamentally damaged or beyond the point of being able to change.

As we listen, we also have the opportunity to attune to their subtle energy movements. For example, when the client loops in thought and clings to their mind, we may be able to see that their energy is concentrated in their head by noticing a density of energy in their forehead. We have the opportunity to map out that subtle energy movement and support the client to be aware of their energy movement. With each thought, there is a correlating subtle energy movement that holds information for the client's transformation. This energy also is part of the map.

In these earlier moments of a session, we also have an opportunity to learn how the client relates to the present moment and their True Self. Are they oriented to the here and now? Do they have access to True Self awareness, or are they hyper-identified with their ordinary mind (Figure 9.1)?

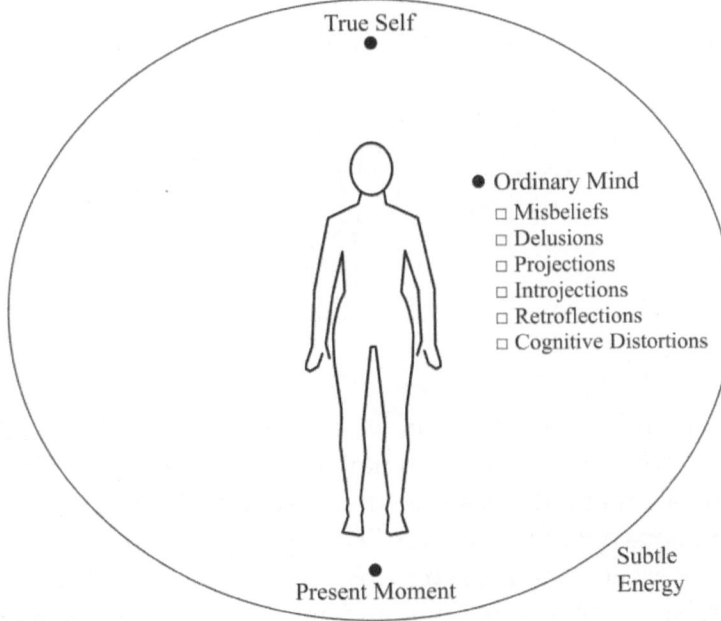

Figure 9.1 Map—Ordinary Mind

As we learn and reflect our client's inner territory, using the awareness continuum helps us to understand the way they relate to their somatic sensations. Do they feel their sensations? Do they analyze their sensations? Are they numb? Are their sensations heightened? Do they orient toward sensations they perceive as negative or positive or both?

In this process of inviting clients into direct experience with their sensations, we gain understanding of their capacity to open to subtle awareness. Have they desensitized from their subtle awareness? Are they attuned to their direct experience? Are they open to increasing this capacity? Do they think their direct experience is irrelevant?

Through deepening our understanding of the client's ordinary mind and subtle awareness, the client's shadow begins to emerge. What lives in their blind spot? What do they disown or reject about themselves? Where are they incongruent? What elements of their inner experience occupy their shadow? The experiences and thoughts that live in the shadow become new landmarks on the map.

When a client clings to their mind and disowns aspects of themselves, their vital force can present as twisted or distorted. By mapping their inner world, we begin to see how the ideas of the ordinary mind relate to the shadow, and how the subtle energy patterns are interconnected between the two (Figure 9.2). Our shared understanding of these inner constructs becomes integral to experiments we co-create (which are explored in later chapters). The very constructs that pull the client off balance become the constructs we follow as the path back home to themselves.

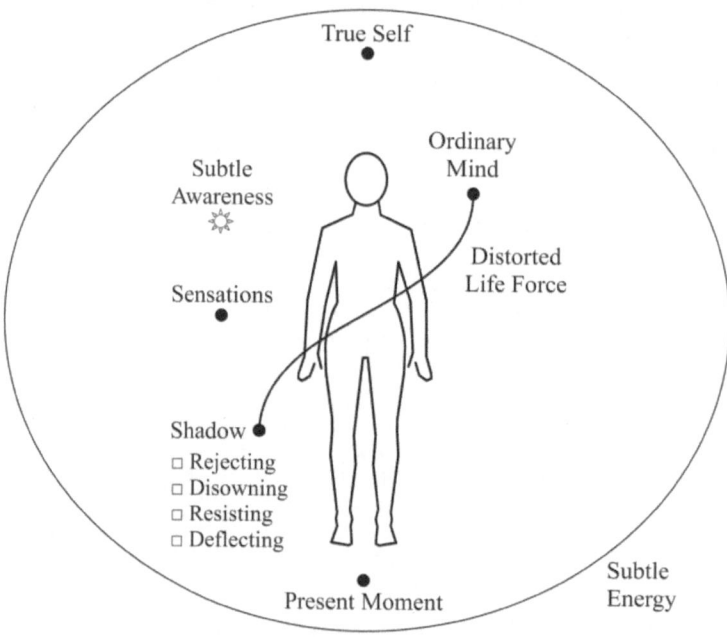

Figure 9.2 Map—Shadow

As the therapeutic work progresses, and we continue to add to our understanding of the client's map, their narratives begin to reveal how they relate to the past and future. Do they cling to the past? Do they regret the past? Do they resent the past? Are they at peace with the past? Do they feel anxious about the future? Do they try to make up stories about what the future holds? Are they excited about the future?

The way they relate to their emotions and intuition also has a marker on the map. What emotions are present? Do they seem overwhelmed by their emotions? Do they resist their emotions? Do they bypass their emotions? Are their emotions heavy, stuck, light, or something else? Are they able to feel and hear their intuition? Do they talk themselves out of their intuition? How does their intuition communicate with them?

Understanding the client's desire is important while learning their map. What the client wants for themselves is the primary guide of the session. Do they know what they want? Are they cut off from their desire? Is their desire an expression of their distortion? Is their desire tied up in wanting others to be different? Do they act in ways that are incongruent with what they want? What part of their pattern do they want to transform?

Similarly, understanding their relationship to their personal power becomes part of the map of their inner territory. Do they give their power away to others? Do they squelch their own power? Do they try to power over others? Do they feel powerless? Is their power distorted?

How they relate with other people and the environment also become part of our understanding of their map. Do they blame other people for how they feel? Do they manipulate and/or control others? Do they think other people are the solution to their inner peace? Are relationships a resource in their life? Do they have resources in their environment? Is the environment they live in safe? Do they have access to nutritious food?

As we learn these various aspects of a client's inner world, we also begin to map out their access to awake awareness (Figure 9.3). When they are in touch with their sensations, emotions, and so on, are they able to lovingly welcome the full range of their experience? Do they have access to self-compassion for their human predicament? With our invitation, are they able to let go of their ordinary mind and shift into an awakened state?

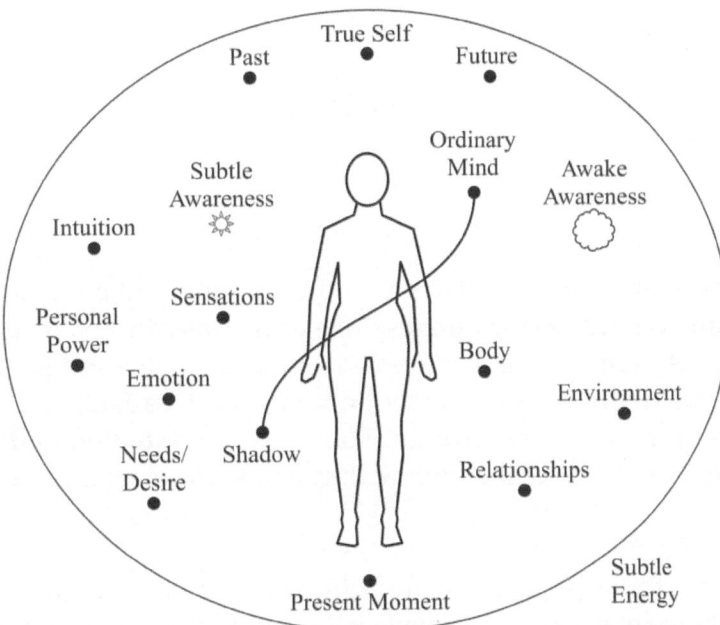

Figure 9.3 Map—Awake Awareness

When we pay attention to the ways in which each landmark pulls a client off center, we are offered insight into the places within the client that need to be illuminated with the light of awareness. These places become the thread we follow as a therapeutic entry point.

For the sake of clarity, Figures 9.1—9.3 showed subtle energy as a large circle. However, when the subtle energy body becomes mistuned by inner distress and unfinished business, the client's presentation isn't quite so clear. The vibrational quality of the subtle energy body is expressed throughout each construct and experience. The appearance of a client's rigid holding patterns permeates their entire subtle energy field.

Each element of their inner landscape relates to all of the other elements. Although each part may appear distinct or separate, a client's inner world is interconnected (Figure 9.4). It is common for clients to look through the lens of one construct and identify with it, and then forget the wholeness of their being. Any perception of fragmentation or brokenness begins to shift once they are seen for the interconnectedness of their experience, for this is where integration begins to unfold.

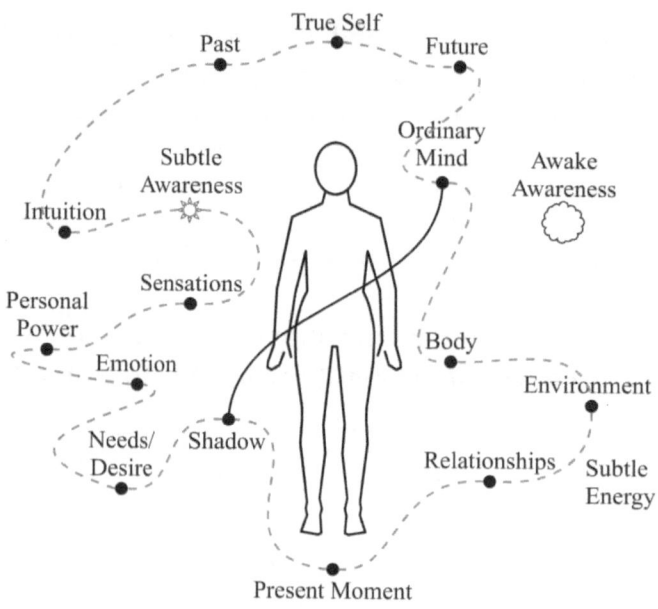

Figure 9.4 Map—Connections

Through our present-centered reflection and attunement, the client is offered a space where they can gain clarity and awareness of various aspects of their inner world that cause them distress. At some point in a session, one aspect emerges as the most accessible to work with. As this distressing construct becomes more salient, it emerges as a figure, and everything else recedes to the ground. Placing more attention and awareness on the figure allows the inner polarity embedded within it to surface, where one inner construct is seemingly opposed to a contrasting construct, causing inner conflict and unrest.

For example, a figure may emerge with the theme of *low self-esteem*. The more present a client becomes with the misbeliefs inherent in this theme, the more two opposing ideas embedded in that theme may emerge: *I'm unlovable* might be opposed to *Nobody is good enough for me*. Mapping out this polarity illuminates for the client the way these ideas keep them off center from themselves (Figure 9.5). Working with a polarity increases awareness as to what unfinished business is guiding a client's habitual patterns. (Working with a polarity is explored in later chapters, along with other potential experiments.)

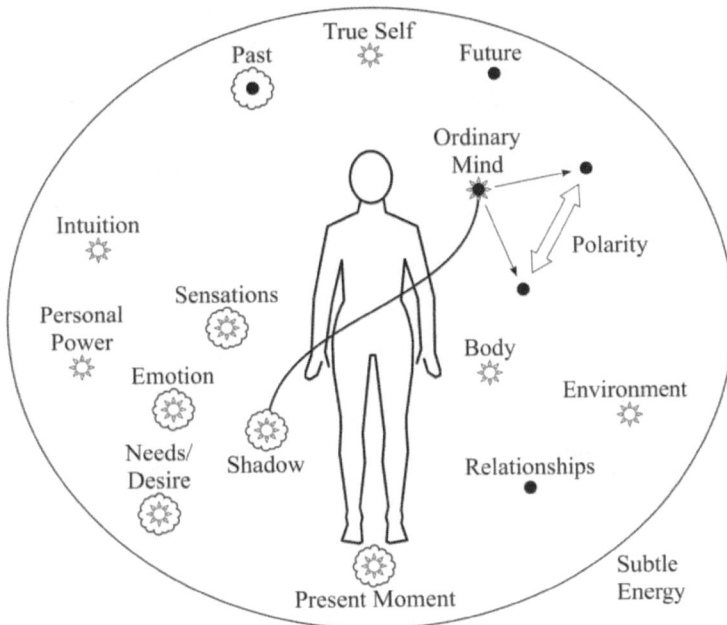

Figure 9.5 Map—Polarity

The process of mapping a client's inner world supports their increasing awareness, which is transformative in and of itself. Through the client's own awareness, emotional processing, nervous system regulation, energetic catharsis, and resolving of unfinished business, the landscape of their inner world begins to transform. In support of this, we also co-create various experiments with our clients, which are creative interventions designed to increase awareness and support integration. Although these experiments can be extremely transformative, we do not *make* integration happen. Our role as a therapist is to be a clear mirror who sees our client's inner map clearly, while also being a guide who can help navigate the map because we have a different vantage point. Integration and alignment are the natural result of the client finding their way through their map while honoring their innate wisdom and spirituality.

As clients become more integrated, aware, and present, the consciousness being held in each element of their inner world is honored. The inherent wisdom embedded in these constructs is acknowledged as the doorway to their transformation. Clients discover and enter into the portal of their transformation through awake awareness. The portal they discover may be in relationship to their power, their body, their emotions, or something else. As they move through their inner territory, they are guided by their innate spirituality as they come back home to their true nature.

Once they enter into the portal of transformation, they begin to find their way through the matrix of their map. Through the work, they become in right relationship with their mind, shadow, emotions, sensations, desire, power, and so on. Guided by their wisdom, they mobilize their emotions, clear subtle energy blocks, access their autonomous power and desire, deepen contact with their body, regulate their nervous system, claim their shadow, and gain clarity of thought. The more aware they become, the more their awake awareness can touch all aspects of them at once (Figure 9.6).

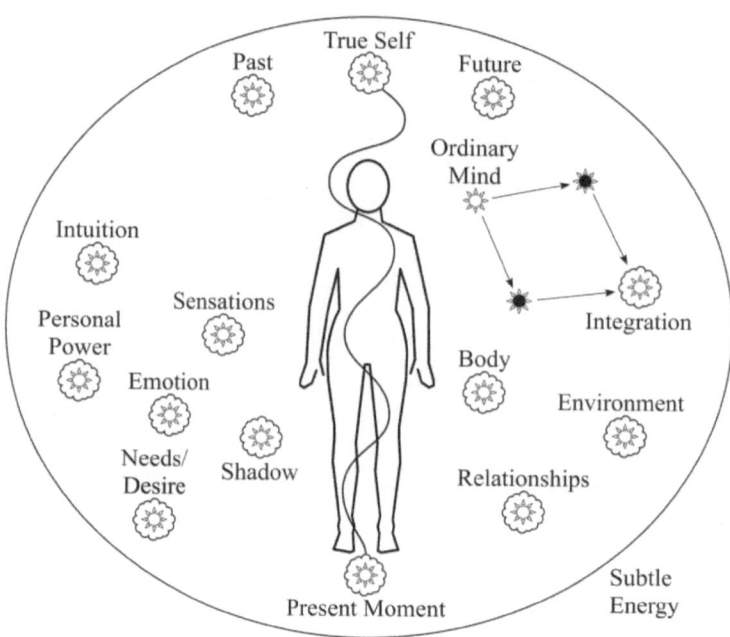

Figure 9.6 Map—Integration

As the client shifts levels of awareness from ordinary to awake, they instinctively find their way back to the core of their being, where their true nature resides. Integrating any aspect that has caused a sense of fragmentation, a client returns to a sense of wholeness. From this place, vitality moves through them spontaneously and without blockages. Their energy body becomes clear and fluffy, and they become the solution to their suffering, where they cultivate internal repair, integration, and autonomy. They leave a session feeling empowered, self-responsible, present, and open to discovering how life unfolds (Figure 9.7).

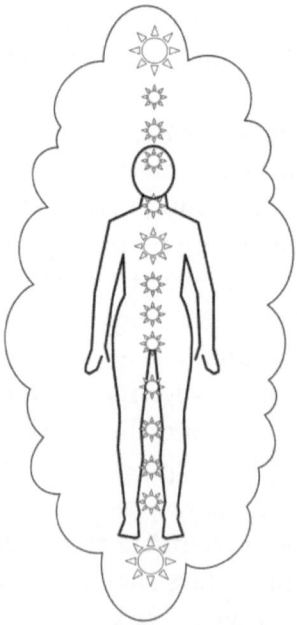

Figure 9.7 Map—Alignment

Questions to Consider When Mapping

All the elements within a person are interconnected. While the person may feel fragmented, we hold the attitude of wholeness and recognize that the whole of the map is greater than the sum of its parts. It is also imperative to trust that subtle awareness (direct experience) and awake awareness (essence of welcoming and love) will alchemize each element into the wholeness of their being.

Here are some questions to consider as you create a map:

♦ **Ordinary Mind:** What delusions, misbeliefs, cognitive distortions, projections, introjections, retroflections, ideas of confluence, and so on pull the attention of their mind? If we distilled the beliefs of the mind down to the essence of their thought, what would it be, and how does the client relate to it?

♦ **Present Moment:** How do they seem to relate to the present moment? Are they fully here in the room? Are they in contact with the here and now?

♦ **Higher Consciousness:** Do they seem regulated and open to their higher consciousness? Do they seem closed off from their Source of love, belonging, compassion, and curiosity?

♦ **Subtle Energy Body:** How does their subtle body appear and feel? Do they seem aware of their subtle self?

♦ **Shadow:** What are the client's blind spots? What do they reject, disown, resist, or deflect about themselves?

♦ **Past:** How do they relate to the past? Do they resent the past? Cling to the past? Accept the past? Bypass the past?

♦ **Future:** How do they relate to the future? Do they anticipate the future with anxiety? Are they hopeful for the future? Do they have longing for the future? Are they afraid they will never change and the future will be like the present?

♦ **Emotions:** What emotions are present and/or persistent? Are they aware of their emotions? How do they relate to their emotions? Are they curious about what their emotions need from them right now?

♦ **Environment:** What environmental factors in the client's home, community, and society are influencing their state of being? Are they aware of these environmental factors? How do they seem to relate to their world outside of the therapy room?

♦ **Relationships:** What significant relationships in the client's life are resources for them? Which ones are drains for them? Do they seem controlling in relationships? Do they seem to let themselves be controlled? Do they long for intimacy? Do they turn away from intimacy? Are they resentful toward others?

♦ **Personal Power:** Are they in touch with their personal power? How do they relate to their personal power? Are their actions congruent with their deepest truth? Do they deceive and misuse power? Do they betray themselves and misuse power?

♦ **Desire:** Do they know what they want? Do they care what other people want? Do they honor their desire? Do they bypass their desire? Do they defer to what others want?

- ♦ **Intuition:** Are they in contact with their intuition? Do they honor their intuition? Do they bypass intuition with fears of the mind?
- ♦ **Subtle Awareness:** How does the client respond when invited into direct experience? Are they able to let go of their thoughts and be with sensation? Can they hear the tone and the words of the sensation? How do they relate to these invitations?
- ♦ **Awake Awareness:** Is the client able to open into awake awareness? Do they genuinely welcome and love their inner distress, or are they clinging to the ordinary mind? Do they feel the magic of their own healing energy? Do they trust their process?

Getting the Lay of the Land

Being in the practice of mapping a client's inner world supports our ability to see them clearly on any given day. It also supports the client's ability to see themselves clearly as they move through life. With a developing sense of self, a client is continually becoming and shifting as they interact with the environment. It's important that we do not put their own map on them, but instead, we stay infinitely curious in each session. Although aspects of their map will again become present, we first open into the present moment I–Thou and see what is relevant in the here and now.

The main skill needed to get the lay of the land is being able to *zoom out*. When we reflect what the client says and how they express themselves, we are zoomed in. We're present and tracking what they say. In these moments, we're learning the client. We're learning how they relate to their thoughts, desires, other people, and so on.

Once we have contactfully gathered sufficient insight into our client's current state, we can zoom out to see the bigger picture of the client's inner territory. When we zoom out, we do not drop contact with the client; we simply contact them in a different way. Where they were once seen and met for their current experience, now they are seen and met for their whole experience.

For example, a client is talking about how they feel in this moment, which is generally a sense of well-being. They continue to say how great they feel, and they relate it to times in their life when they didn't feel great. From a place of being zoomed in, we may reflect that the client feels good in this moment. From a place of being zoomed out, we may map the way they relate to their current experience: "It seems like you're relating to feeling good through the absence of what you don't feel."

How a client relates to each landmark in the map is as important as the landmark itself. This is where awareness is amplified, and the client begins to see their patterns more clearly. The interaction between our awareness and our client's awareness is what allows the map to be accurate. We don't know them as well as they know themselves, and they can't see themselves as clearly as we are able to see them.

As we get the lay of the land, we may use our memory of what's been said at previous sessions as it relates to what is being said now. For example, "I remember you saying this the first time I met you, that you wanted to work in an orphanage." This is highlighting that this desire is persistent, and as such, must be important to who the client is in the world.

We may also receive an intuitive insight into the client's map. This is typically a blind spot of the clients, or it may be the essence of what they are pointing at but remain murky. For example, "I think I'm beginning to learn something about you. It seems like you have a value on reciprocity, and the people in your life may not share that same value." This reflection points to the way a person relates to others, as well as to their own power and desire. This zoomed-out reflection that includes an intuitive guess helps the client to see themselves more clearly. Even if this reflection doesn't fit, it still helps to clarify what is present. For example, the client may say, "Well, yes. I do value reciprocity. But I do have some people in my life that also value that."

Once we have gathered enough insight into the client's map, we can reflect what we think we're seeing. For example, "I see how this would be frustrating: To want connection, and to have your partner say they want that, too, but then to feel alone in the effort to create it." This degree of witness allows a client to see how they move in the world, and from here, they can discover what they truly want for themselves and how they want to meet life. Even when they talk about other people, the work is not to change others or get them to be different. The work is about the client seeing who they are and discovering the deepest, truest way to show up, given the atmosphere of their life.

Maintaining a Sacred Container

To create a sacred container where a client can find their way home to their most awake, resourced Self, we must honor the client and their inner struggle as sacred. It is common for the helping professional to extend their empathy and desire for real change in the client in such a way that they unknowingly cross the sacred boundary. We may even want to carry the burden for the client and help to carry their pain. But, we must remember that this is the client's work to do.

When we hold a sacred container, we come into the deepest contact with our client. We honor them as a whole and see them without judgment. We see them as wise and intuitive and capable of finding their way through the matrix of adaptive strategies and conditioned patterns. We trust their inherent intelligence and ability for organismic self-regulation. We listen to their subtle energy, we welcome their emotions, and we invite their deepest desire into the space.

As we do this, we stay in alignment with the sacred Source of our energy. We regulate our nervous system, and we honor our intuitive senses. We allow the client to process their emotions and energy while we bear witness. We also sense into our empathic experience in our own body while recognizing that this, too, is the client's. With our soul seated in our body, the client has space to find their way back to being seated in themselves. This is what it means to hold a sacred container and meet the client at the sacred boundary.

Lessons from the Therapy Room

I recall a time when I was sitting with a client who had very little access to their body. Guided by a sense of urgency to create change, they followed various trails of thought seeking a solution to their marital struggles. As they put forth this effort, I felt alone in the room, which was a reflection of the client's loneliness. The client was loquacious and seemed to share every thought and idea that came to mind. They were in a marriage that was fraught with deceit, betrayal, and conflict, and they seemed passionate about figuring out how to get their spouse to be a safe space for them.

As I started to map out their *ordinary mind*, some themes that began to emerge included self-loathing, perfectionism, and resentment. The more reflection and co-regulation I offered, the more the client's *shadow* revealed itself as being judgmental and controlling of others. Since they didn't have access to their *sensations*, I would offer reflections such as "You seem to be bracing as you share that." They would cry each time I offered an attuned energetic reflection, saying, "I feel like I am real, like I exist when you see me like that." This became a pin on my map of understanding their subtle awareness, where they had access to it only through my witness.

With my reflection, the client began to deepen into direct experience and accessed *emotions*. Grief around never feeling loved and anger at other people's flaws were present. I learned that they related to their *personal power* by giving their will over to others, and they disowned their *desire* by making others more important than themselves. They bypassed their *intuition* and allowed themselves to be deceived, and they objectified their *body* by ignoring their physical cues. In their *relationships*, they were waiting for the adult to show up while maintaining anger and grief that this hadn't happened in their 50 years of being alive—from others or themselves.

They oriented to the *past* by trying not to be how their parents were and clinging to the loneliness they had felt throughout their life. They feared the *future*, afraid that they wouldn't change and their marriage would stay as it was, or afraid that they would leave and be destitute as they had been in the past.

Although they were challenged to stay *present* in the here and now, they had tremendous access to *awake awareness* and their *True Self*. They were increasingly frustrated that they kept falling into the traps of their mind and leaving this infinite, expansive place that they were quite familiar with. They could not see that their *environment* was not a safe space for them, thus activating their complex trauma responses.

The first experiment I offered was to put the voice of self-loathing in a chair. I did this because they seemed to be most hyper-identified with this sub-personality, and I wanted to support increasing awareness and clarity around what was being held here. When the client saw the voice of self-loathing externalized in the room, they immediately saw the lineage pattern of self-hate. The client's ancestors had been impoverished, and this set off a cycle of internalized oppression passed down through the generations. It took several sessions to untangle this inner voice and distill it down to what aspect of it was theirs to process. At its core, it turned out this voice was a retroflection, where the client hated the way their parents were but had been unable to say that in childhood. Once this self-loathing was directed in the intended way, the client could begin to work with the trauma they had been carrying from childhood into their marriage.

In some ways, this client's map is unchanged, meaning these are the patterns that they identify with and utilize when they are asleep to their True Self. Touched by the light of awareness, however, these patterns are worked with therapeutically, and integration happens on various levels. The work begins by coming into direct experience with sensations, as this capacity guides the depth of what occurs throughout the session. This case is a reminder that healing and repairing the attachment system while actively involved in an unhealthy relationship is extremely challenging, and it takes longer than if the *environment* were a place that nurtured their well-being and health.

Exercise: What's Your Map?

Take this time to consider your own internal map. Remember, this is not to find something to fix about yourself, but an act of increasing self-awareness. As you map out your inner world, consider the following:

- Ordinary Mind: What delusions or misbeliefs do you hold?
- Shadow: What have you disowned or rejected about yourself?
- Body and Sensations: How do you relate to your body and sensations? How do your sensations interact with your thoughts?
- Subtle Energy: How does your subtle energy body feel, move, and express?
- Power: What is your relationship to your power?
- Desire: What is your relationship to your desire?
- Present Moment: How do you relate to the present moment?
- Past and Future: How do you relate to the past and the future?
- Higher Consciousness: Do you have access to your higher consciousness?
- Intuition: How do you relate to your intuition?
- Relationships: How do you relate to your relationships?
- Environment: How do you relate to your environment?

References

Clarkson, P., & Caviccia, S. (2013). *Gestalt counseling in action* (4th ed.). Sage Publications Ltd.

Cole, P. (2022). *The relational heart of Gestalt therapy* (1st ed.). Routledge.

Kaffka, K. (1935). *Principles of Gestalt psychology.* Harcourt, Brace.

Korzybski, A. (1933). *Science and sanity: An introduction to non-aristotelian systems and general semantics.* The Science Press Printing Company.

Mann, D. (2021). *Gestalt therapy: 100 key points and techniques.* Routledge.

Suzuki, S. (1973). *Zen mind, beginner' mind.* Weatherhill Inc.

Zinker, J. (1978). *Creative process in Gestalt therapy* (1st ed.). Vintage.

Deep Transformation

Chapter 10

Creativity and Transformation

When a client's innate spirituality is honored as the catalyst for their transformation, their wisdom collaborates with ours to guide their integration and healing. From a state of present moment awareness, inspiration for creative experimentation organically emerges. The main purpose of an experiment is to increase awareness. However, in the dynamic process of rearranging the therapeutic container and experimenting, many things can happen: A client can mobilize stuck energy, regulate their nervous system, differentiate from their ordinary mind, reclaim the shadow, integrate their polarities, complete unfinished business, and access transpersonal dimensions.

The present moment discovery of how to work with a client's rigid ways of being inspires the creative endeavor of experiments. We creatively invent experiments *with* our clients to invite them into "heightened experience of the body–mind self, authentic encounters with meaningful others, and an impactful relationship with the environment including the [therapist]" (Clarkson & Caviccia, 2013). When the client and the therapist develop experiments together, they do so with the spirit of discovery, as the outcome of an experiment can be neither predicted nor manufactured.

Creativity in therapy provides clients with experiences of how "life can be fully richly lived. This achievable ideal is characterized by acute sensory awareness, a range of emotional responses and effective action" (Clarkson & Caviccia, 2013). This dynamic discovery of change is often "not so much noticed in spoken words as it is in observed enactment" (Brownell, 2010). We can talk with clients for quite some time, and this can be useful to an extent. However, their transformation occurs from the revolutionary act of trying new and different things.

In the presence of our clear witness and the safety of our resonance, clients naturally awaken to their own ego traps and blind spots. For some, these patterns feel like a prison; for others, they feel like barriers to love, inner peace, and empowerment. In any case, clients typically have a genuine desire to find their way through these patterns. As we continue to honor the client's autonomy, we must not make an assumption about what part of their pattern they want to transform. Although it may seem obvious, hearing the client say what they want for themselves ignites the spark of their will. This *spark of will* acts as the guiding light for the transformative work to come. Once the client has named what part of their pattern they are ready to transform, we are ready to collaborate in the creation of an experiment.

DOI: 10.4324/9781003521969-13

Creative Experimentation

Experiments are a truly novel experience designed spontaneously and collaboratively (Zinker, 1978). They are a process by which the client is able to try something that will make the content of their mind more immediately available for experience. There are endless possibilities for experiments, as they give form to the therapeutic content and subsequently create new possibilities (Naranjo, 2004). For example, in an experiment, a client can externalize inner constructs, embodying and speaking from different aspects of their personality. An experiment is also a way to bring environmental factors into the therapy room, such as a person in their life or systems of oppression. They are also a way to bring non-ordinary states into the room, such as dreams and psychedelic journeys.

Experiments support the pillar of phenomenology, where we distinguish experiencing from interpreting or figuring out (Mann, 2021). Instead of talking *about* what they think, the client moves into a unique exploration where they express inherent elements of their experience. We shift the therapeutic container, where we move from *being receptive* to a more *action-oriented* phase. To try something in this way offers a client space to experience the range of their inner and outer worlds, where they familiarize themselves with the authentic expression of their therapeutic content.

As we guide experiments, we prioritize maintaining contact with a client as we co-regulate. Since experiments disrupt homeostasis, nervous system regulation is essential for the learning to unfold organically. As a client naturally mobilizes the stored energy beneath the pattern, they process unfinished business and begin to find their way back home to their true nature. Experiments offer the deepest integration and transformation, which extends well beyond interpreting or reshuffling ideas.

Before we begin an experiment, we must ask the client if they are interested in trying something. Explicitly stating, "Do you want to try something" elicits the consensual nonviolence necessary for transformation to occur. Similarly, the client explicitly saying, "Yes" is necessary to proceed. If the client seems apprehensive, we must pause and ask them what they noticed when they answered. Take time to explore what is true for the client, and do not do an experiment without a clear "Yes."

There is no outline in this approach, as it is a dynamic experience where the client and therapist are in discovery together. By being present and contactful, the creative exploration unfolds naturally. Throughout the experiment, we use a process of trial and error, where we explore new ways of responding rather than reacting. This allows clients an opportunity to see themselves differently, to have a chance to explore possibilities, and to ultimately find enough space from homeostasis that they can explore the concept of choice.

There are no right or wrong answers in an experiment. The learning and the possibilities that unfold are what matters (Wheeler, 2003). Experiments are unique in that clients get an opportunity to confront their habits with compassion as we collaboratively uncover cues in the environment that activate certain patterns. This is often a dynamic, physical enactment that supports mobilizing old energy and releasing past hurt in a safe environment.

Experiments may evoke frustration or stagnancy, and moving through this frustration is important for the client to gain a new understanding and previously unforeseen potential. This newness is experienced as the fertile void, where there are infinite possibilities for the client. As they sit in the infinite, they discover self-responsibility.

Some Things to Consider When Guiding an Experiment

♦ **Get Consent:** The therapist creates a "contract for working," where you get the client's explicit consent that they want to try an experiment.

♦ **Set Context:** Explain to the client what pattern or construct of their map you are observing and how you propose to work with it.

♦ **Be Collaborative:** Check in to see if what you are observing in the client fits for them, and ask them what they think about how you propose to work with it.

♦ **Maintain Contact:** Direct contact with the therapist is more important than *doing* an experiment. As the experiment unfolds, the quality of contact does not change. This is also true for the contact a client has with themselves. Contact remains fundamental throughout the experiment, and it will likely deepen as well.

♦ **Be Direct:** Once the experiment begins, the therapist becomes more directive while also maintaining contact via the awareness continuum, reflective listening, and attunement. Since a client will not know how to navigate this on their own, your direction is necessary throughout an experiment.

♦ **Be Present:** Experiments are present moment centered and invite the client into immediate access to what is already available within them. It is not a role play.

♦ **Phenomenology:** An experiment invites the client to actively embody their thoughts/emotions/impulses and express them as they arise rather than avoiding them or analyzing them.

♦ **Subtle Energy:** Attuning to the subtle energy field throughout an experiment makes for a potent and transformative process. For example, when a client gets space from an inner construct, support them in fully getting the energy of that construct in the other chair. Have them feel into their energy now that they have space.

♦ **Tangible Access:** Experiments bring the therapeutic content into the room in a more tangible way. Instead of analyzing or rearranging ideas, the therapist shifts the therapeutic environment via experiments as a way to bring the client more fully into the here and now.

♦ **Increase Awareness:** An experiment is always relevant to what's in the room, which may be aspects of a client's conditioned self, a younger self, or someone else from their life. The learning that unfolds cannot be achieved through traditional talk therapy.

♦ **Therapeutic Surrender:** The directive nature of experiments allows the client to surrender and make deeper contact with aspects of self. It's not the type of directive where I know better than you, so you do what I say. It's guiding them in the places that have previously been unfinished and in their blind spots.

Types of Experiments

♦ **Explication or Translation:** Inviting the client to translate nonverbal experiences, sensations, and expressions into words. For example, "If anger had a voice, what would it say?" or "If (this sensation/movement/tears) had a voice, what would it say?" By making implicit content explicit, the client has the opportunity to deepen into the phenomenology of their experience and listen to the wisdom of their current lived experience.

♦ **Expressive Techniques:** Asking the client to *exaggerate* a specific behavior, motion, or emotion. This allows a client to follow impulses and desires of the moment, which allows intensification. For example, invite the client to exaggerate their indirectness, control, self-criticism, etc. "You never overcome anything by resisting it. You only overcome anything by going deeper into it" (Naranjo, 2004). Alternatively, you can ask them to *increase the volume* and say something louder and with more energy or to *repeat* a specific behavior, motion, or emotion.

♦ **Suppressive Techniques:** Eliminating something that inhibits contact and moves them away from the present. "Instead of looping in the infertile torrent of preoccupations that lead them nowhere, we invite them to experience the moment and feel instead" (Perls, 1973). Stop doing what they're doing and notice what that's like. For example, asking them to notice what happens when they stop fidgeting.

♦ **Integrative Techniques:** Integration of personality is explored through the intra-psychic dialogue. Two-chair is the most common integrative technique, as it offers a place to synthesize different elements of a client's psyche that are in conflict. Through our observations and suggestions, the client is guided to clearly separate two aspects of the conditioned self and externalize them in the room by placing them in two different chairs. Moving back and forth between two chairs, we guide the client to embody both parts of the personality. This allows aspects of their psyche to directly communicate with one another, which increases consciousness. We will explore it in detail in Chapter 11, "Working with Polarities." Integrative techniques can also be done internally with visualization; however, learning two-chair experiments first makes visualizations more effective.

♦ **Completing Unfinished Business:** Empty chair is the most common technique to complete unfinished business. By bringing in the energy of a person or an establishment and placing it in an empty chair, a client can process and heal unfinished business. By giving form to the consciousness of the other person or people, a client has the opportunity to process their authentic expression as it relates to them. Examples of empty chair include bringing in a person who ghosted them, inviting in their ancestors, or bringing in the establishment that they feel oppressed by.

♦ **Reparenting:** The work of reparenting supports clients in healing their attachment wounds, clearing introjections, and creating a secure base with themselves. A younger aspect of the client can be brought into the room via the empty chair technique or explored with visualization. (This will be explored in more detail in Chapter 12

Being Receptive and Being Directive

The skills of holding sacred space are primarily receptive skills, where we find resonance with the client and meet them where they are. Rather than instructing a client what to do, we are simply *being with* them. This quality of receptivity and resonance cultivates safety and awareness, which is necessary to foster before moving into an experiment.

Experiments are directive in nature. Direction is important for an experiment because we are guiding a client through the exploration. A client would not know how to move through an experiment on their own, and our directives will support them in finding their way. When the quality of contact is sufficient, and the client says "yes" to the experiment, our attuned and mindful direction is a welcome relief to support them in finding their way through the matrix of their inner territory. However, we continue to attune and collaborate as we navigate the experiment.

Below is a list of receptive skills and directive skills. Over time, we weave them together in a skillful dance of attuned contact and disrupting homeostasis.

Receptive Skills

♦ **Seeing a client's wholeness:** Trust in a client's inherent movement toward health and honor their wisdom.
♦ **Reflective listening:** Repeat their words back to them.
♦ **Empathetic listening:** Listening for the deeper emotion and need. Summarize what you think you're learning about them.
♦ **Empathetic witnessing:** Attuning to the emotional body. Letting them know how they seem ("You seem …").
♦ **Energetic witnessing:** Tracking the subtle energy body.
♦ **Pausing for raw emotions:** Sitting in silence.
♦ **Feeling into your body:** Find resonance in your body and listen to the sensations you feel in their presence.
♦ **Trying on what it's like to be them:** "I imagine …" or "It sounds like …."
♦ **Letting them know how you feel in their presence:** Use this skill sparingly to increase contact and give voice to the way you are affected by a client. "I feel my feet on the ground when you say that. What do you notice?"

Directive Skills

♦ **Awareness continuum:** This is gentle directive, bringing attention into the here and now.
♦ **Directing breath:** Telling the client to notice where their breath does move and let go of the exhale is an attuned directive.

- **Directing attention:** When a client has moved past an idea or memory, you can bring attention back to it: "I have attention on …."
- **Directing energy:** When a client notices blocked energy, invite them to wrap it in awareness and ask it what it needs.
- **Asking them to close their eyes:** In order to increase their interoceptive sense of their inner landscape, you may want to invite them to close their eyes, then ask, "What do you notice as you turn toward yourself?"
- **Experiments:** In a two-chair, you may tell a client when to switch seats. You may tell them to say something to the other chair and see what they notice. With an expressive experiment, you may tell a client, "Do that movement with your arms again," or "Say that louder." These directives are in service of increasing awareness and disrupting homeostasis.

Sitting at an Impasse

At some point during an experiment, a client will likely meet an impasse, where they are preventing themselves from moving through unfinished business (Perls, 1973). When the client seems trapped and attached to their perspective, the energy in the therapeutic process feels sterile, as if growth cannot occur here.

An impasse may be expressed as the client talking a lot. Staying at the level of the ordinary mind, the client may talk about themselves to try to figure themselves out or talk themselves into a new experience. Alternatively, an impasse may be expressed as moments of dullness or too much silence. The client may feel lost and unsure of what to do or how to be.

Other expressions of an impasse include confusion, frustration, guilt, blame, or deep grief. Any trap set by the mind that has the client feel imprisoned by their own way of being is an impasse. In these moments, we must tend to the impasse as sacred. Knowing that all behavior is adaptive, we must also trust the wisdom of the impasse.

If we do not honor the impasse, but instead, we try to fix it or change it in some way, we are becoming induced into our client's sense of powerlessness. To stay awake in these moments and fully trust our client's ability to find their way through, while also maintaining contact, is an affirmation of our client's wisdom and ability. There are infinite opportunities to increase awareness in these sterile moments that become the guiding light for finding their way through the matrix of their inner map.

Here are some inquiries for you to consider about what arises within you as the client encounters an impasse:

- How do you feel when a client is at an impasse?
- How do you feel in moments of silence?
- What insight or wisdom is present in the impasse?
- What insight or wisdom is present in the dullness?

- How can you support the increasing of awareness with clients who are stuck at an impasse?
- How can your own awake awareness support the resolution of the impasse?

Cycle of Therapeutic Transformation

The cycle of therapeutic transformation (depicted in Figure 10.1) begins with increasing awareness through attunement and reflections. In these early stages of the therapeutic transformation, we contact the client as they are and support them to be mindful of how they feel and what they think. As we become present with the client, we invite awareness to guide the session by asking present moment/open questions.

Our empathetic listening creates space to gain understanding of the client's inner world. As a clear mirror of reflection, the client sees themselves more clearly through our neutral witness. Discovering the map of the client's subjective experience requires that we zoom out to see the bigger picture of how they disrupt contact with themselves, the present moment, and their environment.

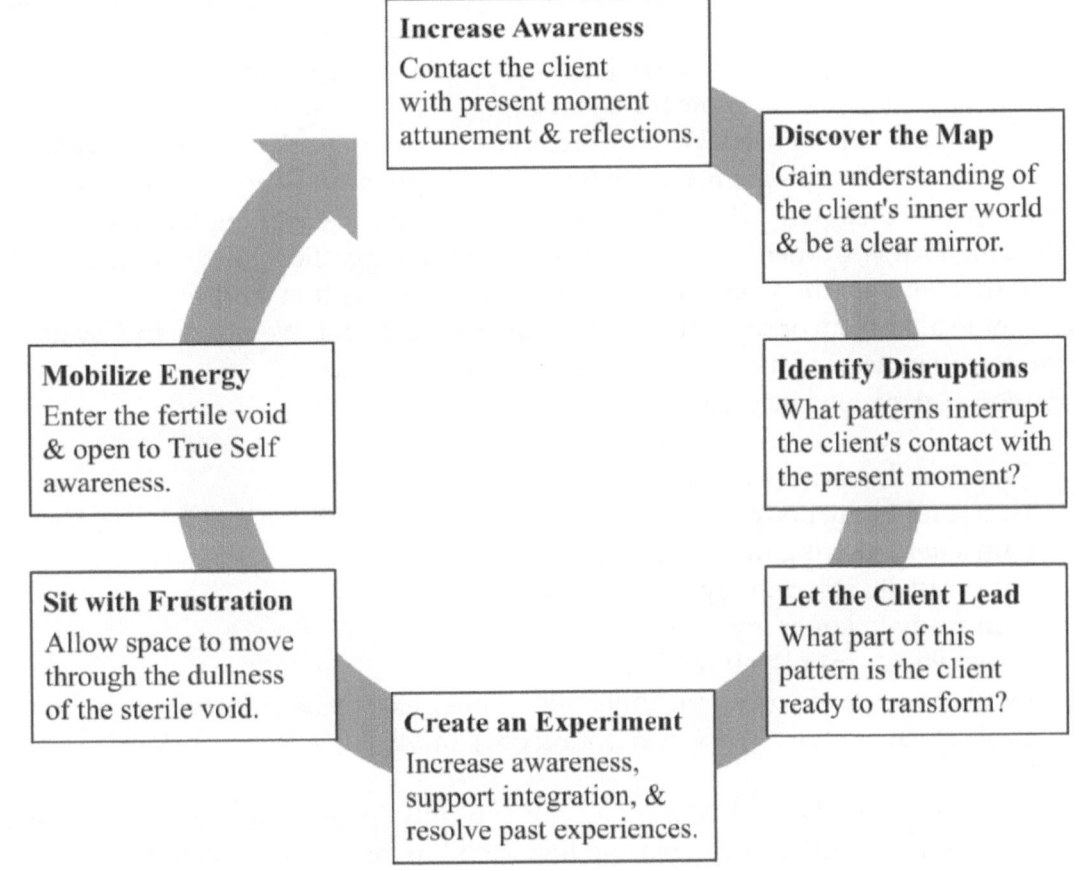

Figure 10.1 Therapeutic Cycle

As we map out their inner world, we begin to identify the patterned ways of being that cause the client to disrupt contact with the present moment. Recognizing contact disruptions is less about the language of contact boundary disturbances and more about ideas and behaviors that the client is hyper-identified with and that cause them distress. In these disruptions, we may discover a polarity, unfinished business, or some other construct that becomes the figure of our therapeutic work.

At this point, our receptive presence has created safety and resonance in the container. Before we move forward into the action phase of the session, we need to allow the client to lead where they go next. Asking them what they want for themselves or what part of this pattern they are ready to transform guides what happens next.

Next, we can co-create an experience with the client. Our collaborative creativity serves to increase awareness, support integration, and resolve unfinished business. We set up a contract for working by asking the client if they are open to trying something. When the client has a clear "yes" to the experiment, we have their consent to proceed, and we explore confronting rigid habits and patterns with compassion.

As we guide the client through the experiment, they have an opportunity to feel their frustration with themselves. Since their patterns were created to support them in finding safety when the environment was unable to meet their needs, they may meet their own inner resistance to change. We pause for the raw emotions and sit in silence when appropriate. Silence is a sacred pause that honors the client's experience deeply.

Continuing with the experiment, energy mobilizes, and catharsis happens naturally. This type of catharsis occurs because awareness has saturated their inner experience, making room for anything that is ready to move to release. Once catharsis happens, the client is able to find their way into full contact with themselves and embody their true nature. They discover the infinite possibilities of the fertile void and come into an expression of true autonomy.

To close the cycle, we may invite the client to give language to what is true for them now, given what they just experienced. We may even offer some suggestions based on what we just learned about them. These statements are framed as affirmations, and once the client speaks the words, we ask them what they notice in their body. We are looking for full congruence and full resonance with their words. When we offer a suggestion for the affirmation, it is important that we own the words as coming from our perception, and that we make room for the client to alter them or say something completely different. We can do this by using the sentence stem "I'm hearing it as …" or "I think I'm hearing it as …."

Common affirmations include:

+ "I am safer honoring myself."
+ "I am safer in my body."
+ "I am safer speaking my truth."
+ "I am ready to stand in my power."
+ "I am ready to honor my heart."
+ "I deserve to treat myself with respect."
+ "I will always love you (to the inner young one), exactly as you are."
+ "I will always cherish you (inner young one) and listen to your wisdom."

In a 50-minute session, the first 20 minutes are typically focused on awareness, mapping, identifying an inner conflict, and exploring distorted life force. Co-regulation is interwoven throughout. When the experiment begins, the client deepens into contact and moves through the sterile void and into the fertile void in the last 30 minutes.

Not every session has a therapeutic cycle. Oftentimes, there is tremendous value in simply listening and co-regulating. There is immense value in reflecting and supporting a client's clarity. When the client is ready to shift the patterns that hold them back or cause them distress, we offer them a new way to explore themselves. Clients are ready to deepen into contact at different points during a working relationship.

Lessons from the Therapy Room

Being a therapist is sacred work, where I get to sit with clients in their raw and tender emotions. As they find their way through their pain, struggle, and ego, I have the honor to witness the Divine in action when they discover the path back to themselves. It is a holy moment of pure embodiment.

Earlier in my career, I was afraid that I would break contact with a client if I became more directive. For me, being with clients in their pain and listening deeply is a natural way to hold space. However, at some point, sessions became dull and lackluster. Too much listening proved to be uninspiring of change.

Given the history from which gestalt therapy was created, I wanted to find my own language and my own way to be directive. I wanted to be nonviolent, consensual, and collaborative. My directives became *invitations*, where I invited the client to try something and asked them what they thought. "If you're open to trying this, I'd like to invite you to …." I felt much more at ease with this language, and it gave me space to find my way in directing experiments.

Asking a client what part of their pattern they were ready to transform was a revolutionary moment in my career. I realized that the client's desire was the guide in their experiment. With this epiphany, I also realized that my desire, combined with the client's, was a point of contact. If I didn't have access to my desire, I couldn't direct an experiment. To be directive, knowing what I want and what the client wants, is necessary; otherwise, I had no instructions for what to do next. Being willing to let go of my desire if the client discovered they wanted something else for themselves ensured that I was not holding an agenda.

With practice, I learned to meet the client at the sacred boundary and fully trust their inherent wisdom. I was astonished by the deep work clients were able to do when they were trusted and honored in this deep way. Since I, myself, had never experienced this level of repair in psychotherapy, I wasn't sure it was possible. However, now that I have facilitated this deep transformative work for over a decade *and* teach students how to lead in this way, I feel excited for the paradigm shift that is happening in the field of mental health healing.

Exercise: Create an Experiment for Yourself

Now that you've mapped out your patterns, choose one aspect of yourself that you are ready to transform. Create an experiment in service of your own transformation.

For example, if you notice that your ordinary mind judges your appearance, you may create a mirror exercise for yourself. Set the timer for 5 min, look yourself straight in the eyes, and tell yourself the truth about who you really are. Update the old narrative with True Self-talk.

Another example might be if you noticed your relationship to other people is to prioritize them as important. You might set up a social experiment for yourself, and the next time you are at a social event, ask at least three people to do something for you. Let yourself really receive from others.

I encourage you to contact what comes up as you read this now. Is there excitement? Resistance? Something else? Contact and trust that the process of deeper knowing of your True Self is worth the time to explore and understand. After the experiment, make time to reflect on the experience.

References

Brownell, P. (2010). Spirituality in the praxis of gestalt therapy. In J. H. Ellens (Ed.), *The healing power of spirituality: How faith helps humans thrive* (pp. 93–103) (Vol. 3). Routledge/Taylor & Francis Group.

Clarkson, P., & Caviccia, S. (2013). *Gestalt counseling in action* (4th ed.). Sage Publications Ltd.

Mann, D. (2021). *Gestalt therapy: 100 key points and techniques*. Routledge.

Naranjo, C. (2004). *Gestalt therapy: The attitude and practice of an atheoretical experientialism.* Crown House Pub Ltd.

Perls, F. (1973). *The Gestalt approach and eye witness to therapy* (1st ed.). Science and Behavior Books, Inc.

Wheeler, G. (2003). Contact and Creativity: The Gestalt Cycle in Context. In M. S. Lobb & N. Amendt-Lyon (Eds.), *Creative License* (pp. 163–178). Springer, Vienna.

Zinker, J. (1978). *Creative process in Gestalt therapy* (1st ed.). Vintage.

Chapter 11

Working with Polarities

As two seemingly opposing energies, polarities are expressed through habits of the personality that cause a client distress. Internal polarities begin to form when the personality is developing in childhood. The personality forms quietly, in the privacy of one's mind, in relationship to one's environment, which includes other individuals and the psychic field (Lewin, 1935). In the presence of misattuned, neglectful, or abusive caregivers, psychic tensions arise, creating internal contradictions, or *polarities*.

When the environment consistently fails to meet a child's needs for safety, connection, trust, and attunement, the child feels a sense of shame for not having their needs met (Heller & LaPierre, 2012). As the child attempts to make sense of the failure of their caregivers, they develop an identity that reflects the *ideal* of how they want to be seen, where anything that they believe makes them unlovable is pushed into the shadow. The psychic tensions between a person's *primary strategies* of their ideal self and the *shadow strategies* of their disowned parts are attempting to discharge energy, mobilizing them into action to try to get their needs met.

The mutually dependent factors of the personality and the environment are viewed as a functional part of the situation (Foschi & Lombardo, 2006). The child finds a way to create a sense of belonging and safety through the primary strategies and shadow (or shame-based) strategies developed in an environment not designed for their well-being.

As the child grows into an adult, what was once functional becomes a habit of the personality. A person's mental processes are viewed as part of the totality of their central nervous system processes, which has "phenomenal properties and constitutes consciousness" (Lindorfer, 2020). When unresolved experiences from the past persist in the phenomenology and consciousness of the client, the current field they exist within becomes the environment in which they try to discharge their inner polarities. As we begin to work with their polarities in a session, they are able to access the phenomenology and consciousness being held in their internal contradictions.

In a therapeutic session, the therapist is now part of the environment the client exists within. Our presence and attunement create an opening for a client's polarities to naturally emerge. There is no need to search or dig for a client's polarity. Instead, we allow it to come forth organically, without agenda. As part of the psychic field, we have the opportunity to create an experience with the client where they can move through their polarity and discover their way back into alignment.

DOI: 10.4324/9781003521969-14

Common Missteps When Working with a Polarity

There are four common missteps clinicians might make when working with polarities. The first common misstep is mistaking an aspect of health as part of the polarity. For example, a therapist may think the polarity is between a client's sense of feeling lost and their wisdom. However, a person's wisdom does not block energy unless it is propaganda that they are using to bypass their experience. The true polarity would be between the *voice of confusion* (lost) and the voice of *I shouldn't feel this way* (propaganda disguised as wisdom). Alternatively, the polarity may be between the *voice of confusion* (lost) and the *voice of rigid ideals* (unyielding desire disguised as wisdom).

The second common misstep is to ignore the phenomenology of the polarity and focus only on talking *about* each construct. When a therapist fails to invite the client into deeper contact and awareness of their inner mind–body connection, there are missed opportunities to unblend the polarity, regulate the nervous system, and work with the subtle energy present. Staying with the phenomenology of each aspect of the polarity makes working with it more effective, integrative, and cathartic.

The third common misstep is to use two sensations in the body as the polarity. When a client presents with two felt sense experiences that are seemingly opposing one another, it's important to be curious about how these sensations relate to their thought patterns. Discovering what thought processes correspond with each body sensation allows the wisdom of the way the body is holding the polarity to have a voice. The consciousness of the polarity lives in the mind–body connection. Ignoring the body bypasses phenomenology, and ignoring the mind bypasses personality habits that need to be understood.

Lastly, the fourth common misstep is when a therapist prioritizes contact between themselves and the client, as opposed to the client being in contact with the elements of the polarity. The beauty of working with polarities is that the client engages in a dialogue between opposing aspects of their inner world. Clients will often turn to the therapist and tell us what they think about the other part, which is fine as long as the therapist listens and invites the client to tell that to the other subpersonality. By staying in communication with their own inner process, the client is more likely to naturally integrate what has historically been fragmented. Where contact between therapist and client was once an important focus, this relationship recedes as the client explores deepening into contact with themselves.

Unblending Polarities

Before a polarity has been identified, it lives within the client's psyche as an inner conflict or pattern that causes distress. When these two opposing constructs are blended together, they seem big and insurmountable to the ordinary mind. The client may feel contracted around their inner polarity or resist it with the force of self-judgment. The process of unblending a polarity allows the client to get space from the polarity as well as to create more distance between the aspects of the polarity.

Inner spaciousness is an expression of increased awareness (Siegel, 2010). The more space a client has from their polarity, the more they elevate their consciousness in relationship to that polarity. Similarly, the more space each aspect of the polarity has from the other, the more consciousness the client has in relationship to each aspect.

Here are some ways to help clients unblend their polarities:

- Invite your client to put an aspect of the polarity in a chair or cushion. Direct them to use their hands, words, breath, and movement to get all of the energy of this aspect over on the chair. This supports unblending the subtle energy of the polarity, which can be extremely regulating and clarifying.
- Demonstrate with your own body the moving of the aspect into the other chair. Your presence in the phenomenology helps to unblend the energy.
- Invite your client to imagine an aspect of the polarity as if it were sitting in front of them. Have them focus on the aspect of the polarity and see its energetic expression.
- Ask your client how they feel once they have space from the other aspect. Invite them into the phenomenology of the seat they are sitting in as they sense into the space created from unblending.
- Ask them how the other aspect seems from this vantage point. Invite them to share the size, shape, color, or texture of the appearance of the other aspect. This supports their mind in differentiating from this part of the personality.
- Invite them to speak directly to the other part of the polarity from the aspect they are embodying. In this step, the thinker becomes the thought; the feeler becomes the feeling. Paradoxically, by becoming what they resist, they are better able to unblend and differentiate from aspects of the psyche.
- Invite them to switch seats and notice the energetic difference. Support them in accessing the phenomenology of this new chair.
- Remind them what the other aspect said to them. This helps them to process each part as separate. Ask them what they notice when they hear that or if there is anything they want to say back.
- Move slowly to allow nervous system regulation and deepening into each part.
- Once the polarity seems unblended, try moving faster to keep them unblended. If the client begins to speak on behalf of the other part, ask them to move to the other seat.

Two-Chair Polarity Exercise

Because one aspect of the polarity is in the forefront of a client's ordinary awareness, and the other is seated in their shadow, externalizing these inner constructs allows the client to see them more clearly. Two-chair experiments are well known in gestalt because they illustrate the power of getting space from constructs of the mind, making it possible to increase levels of awareness and work with them consciously.

Two-chair experiments make it possible for a client to see the way that their inner world has been organized around unmet needs from the past. As they move through the experiment, they have the opportunity to clear introjections, which are messages acquired from other people, and give themselves what they've always needed. They express their deepest truth, listen to themselves deeply, and find their way into an integrated sense of Self.

The shadow or exiled aspect of the polarity has the opportunity to speak what's true for the consciousness of this characteristic. Instead of repressing or fighting with their shadow, the client embodies it and gives it a voice. This is a very regulating experience because it fosters congruence, where the client has more integrity and alignment. In this process, clients regulate their nervous system, move blocked energy, and open to themselves. When complete, the client enters into the fertile void, where there are infinite possibilities and deep self-responsibility.

Here is the evolution of a two-chair experiment:

Once the poles are identified, and it is known that they are opposing one another, ask the client if they are open to trying an experiment. If they have a clear "yes," proceed.

Set a framework for working by telling the client what you are inviting them to do. Invite the client to put one aspect of the polarity in a different chair. As they put one aspect into the chair, invite them to use their hands, scoop up the energy of that aspect, and literally place it in the other chair until all the energy of that aspect is in the other chair. Have them say it aloud: "I am putting (name of the aspect) into that chair over there."

Once complete, invite the client to take a few breaths and notice how they feel on getting space from the other aspect. Then, ask the client how the other aspect seems to them, which helps them to unblend even more. Then, ask the client if there is anything they want to say to it. Whatever they say is welcome, but help them to phrase it in the first person and speak directly to the other aspect, and then ask them what they notice when they say that, to support the awareness continuum.

Have the client stay in this one seat as long as they need to get to the deeper facets of their psyche and subtle energy, and then have them switch. Once they switch seats, have them feel into the energy of the new chair. Ask them what they notice. Next, reflect what the other aspect said to them, summarizing what was said from the other part. Ask the client what they notice as they hear this and what they would like to say to the other part. This gives the client an opportunity to embody and speak from their shadow. For example, they may say, "I love being overwhelmed. It makes me feel important," or "I like being alone. I feel safe when I'm alone," or "I like being overweight. No one can hurt me when I'm protected like this."

It is important to note that if the client says, "Nothing. I can't even talk to that part," have them say that to the other part. For example, "Tell that to that part, 'I have nothing to say to you.'" This keeps the communication going and supports moving through an impasse.

Continue to facilitate a conversation between the polarities, having the client switch back and forth between seats. Be directive and contactful. Once both aspects have been heard, and collaboration has begun, have the client take a third seat, the seat of awake awareness. From this vantage point, have the client look at the polarity and share how they seem. Ask them if there is anything they want to say to them.

Then, invite them to bring the two aspects back into them, in the proportion that they want and in the place that they want.

Because there are so many unknowns, it is important to remember that we are not the expert. We are the witness, the mirror. And once the landscape begins to change through the experiment, we're still mapping out the way the client relates to themselves. We are co-creating with the client, and we are learning along with them. Every time is a fresh, new experiment with infinite unknowns. This is, in part, what makes this work so dynamic and profound.

Outline for Facilitating a Two-Chair Experiment

1. **Get consent:** Do you want to try something?
2. **Identify the polarity:** Reflect the pattern you are hearing/seeing, and ask the client if this fits for them.
3. **Confirm the names of the polarity:** "Is this what you would call them? Or is there something else that fits better?"
4. **Set Context:** Once the pattern is identified, explain to the client what you'd like to do: "I'm wanting to invite you to do an experiment where these two aspects/parts have the opportunity to communicate."
5. **Re-check consent:** How does that sound?
6. **Start the experiment:** "The chair you are sitting in will be the voice of _____. And I'd like to invite you to put the voice of _____ in that chair."
7. **Direct the experiment:** Be creative and maintain contact as you guide the process.
    a. Invite the client to put one aspect in the other chair. They can use their hands and their words as they get all of the energy of that one aspect in the other chair.
    b. Ask them what they notice in their body on getting space from the other aspect.
    c. Ask them how the other aspect seems to them.
    d. Ask them if there is anything they want to say to the other chair.
    e. Reflect and ask them what they notice in their body.
    f. Ask if there is anything else they want to say.
    g. Eventually, tell them you're going to ask them to switch chairs, and ask them what they notice what you say that.
    h. If they're okay with that, have them move chairs.
    i. Once they switch, ask them what they notice in their body in this new chair.
    j. Remind them what the other aspect said.
    k. Ask them if there is anything they want to say to the other chair.
    l. Reflect and ask them what they notice in their body.
    m. Ask if there is anything else they want to say.
8. **Switch back and forth:** Have the client switch from chair to chair as you facilitate the communication. Invite the client to sense into their body as they access the deeper truth of their experience.
9. **Have them take a third seat:** Once each chair is feeling heard, and they are collaborating, invite the client to take a third seat, that of the conscious witness.
    a. Ask them how these two aspects seem from here.
    b. Ask them if there is anything they want to say to them.
    c. Then, ask them to invite them back in as they are now, heard, seen, and transmuted.

Somatic Integration

When we work with polarities, we are focusing on two opposing constructs of the client's inner world; however, we are working with the client's whole being. Their ego, shadow, emotions, nervous system, attachment system, subtle energy, innate spirituality, and more are being accessed as they move through the experiment. *Somatic integration* is a wonderful way to work with polarities in a dynamic and embodied way.

Drawing on expressive and suppressive techniques, somatic integration offers a client the opportunity to feel the way through their polarities and back to their midline. The felt experience of a polarity is emphasized through expression and suppression, while the client speaks from the various elements of the polarity. In this experiment, a client stays in one seat, and the polarities are unblended through the movements of expression and suppression.

In general, the aspect of the client's ego that they feel most identified with is what is amplified with the expressive technique. With their words and their body, the client exaggerates the message of the ego. They repeat this and continue to feel the way their body holds this aspect of the polarity. After a few minutes, the client takes the shape of the shame-based identification that lives in the unconscious mind. They get small and contained as they speak from this exiled aspect of themselves.

For example, a client may be talking about their imposter syndrome, explaining the way they feel insecure even though they are an expert in their field. As they speak about this, we are noticing their physical movements, where they get stronger and bigger when they talk about being an expert, and they shrink when they talk about their insecurities. With our attuned presence, we would reflect the polarity we think we are seeing: "It sounds like you know you're an expert, yet you feel like you're not enough." If this reflection fits for the client, we would then ask them if they would like to try something.

If the client is open to trying an experiment, we ask them to take the shape of the expert. With their whole body and their words, express how they are one of the best in their field. The client may open their arms and speak more loudly, and we encourage them to continue to express this feeling of being the best and repeat their words.

After a few minutes, we then direct the client to move into the shape of insecurity. With their whole body and their words, have them contain themselves with the feelings of self-doubt. The client may get really small and say they feel like hiding under a rock. We encourage them to continue to contain their energy and feel the way insecurity is being held in their body as they repeat the words of self-doubt.

After a few minutes, have them move into the expression of being the expert. With their whole body and their words, have them exaggerate this pride. And then, direct them back into the expression of self-doubt. With their words and their body, have them speak from self-doubt.

Going back and forth a few times with their words and their body shape helps the client to contact different aspects of this polarity. After a few times, have the client only take the shape of each side of the polarity whilespeaking the words. Invite them to breathe and feel into their experience. First, have them move quickly through the polarity. Then, have them slow down and move through the polarity. Because the vagus nerve is impacted by the somatic holding of the polarity, the client may feel a bit disoriented as they reset their nervous system.

Once sufficient energy has been mobilized, have the client sense into the way to the midline between these polarities. With their body moving back and forth between the polarities, have them discover for themselves the shape of the midline. Once they find that midline, have them speak from what is true here. A client may say, "I am here to offer my gifts, and I cannot control how they are received." Invite them to take a few breaths and feel this in their body, and then repeat the words a few times to anchor into their midline.

This profound experiment touches all aspects of a person's being, as it preferences phenomenology rather than thoughts and interpretation.

Visualization

Where two-chair gives voice to the different aspects of the polarity, somatic integration prioritizes the felt sense. Visualization varies from this in that it supports the client in seeing themselves with their metaphysical eyes. With their eyes closed, we invite the client to bring their attention to the voice of the most dominant energy of the polarity. As if it were sitting in front of them, ask the client how it seems to them. How does it look? How big is it? What is the energy it is holding?

If a client is working with an antagonistic retroflection, for example, they may be looking at the voice of the inner critic. A client may see the energetic appearance of this retroflection as scared and fragile. Have them continue to see this aspect in their mind's eye, for the more they can see it, the more awareness they have in relationship to it. Ask them what that scared and fragile look is like, getting a good sense of the energetic expression of this construct. They might say, "Restless and wiry."

Once they can see it, have them see it from their witness mind, "I see you. I see that you feel scared and restless." This supports the differentiation and disruption of homeostasis. Then, ask them if there is anything they want to say to this aspect. For example, they may say, "You're taking over everything. I can't feel at peace when you're here." This indicates inner resistance and is an indicator as to why the polarity exists. Next, ask them what they notice when they say that.

What they feel in their body as they speak to the aspect of the polarity is an indicator of what is being polarized. For example, if the client says, "I feel hopeless. Like I want to give up. What's the point? It's always going to have control," we have an indicator that the polarity is between restlessness and hopelessness. These are two opposing forces that are blocking energy. Ask them what they notice when they express this. Then, ask them if there is anything that they need from the other aspect of the polarity (from restlessness in this case). "I need you to trust me," they may say.

Facilitate a conversation between the two aspects, where the feelings and needs of both sides of the polarity are spoken and honored. As this is all taking place, attune to the subtle energy in the body, follow the client's energy, and support the mobilization of energetic blocks. This is a very simple and approachable intervention that supports clients in increasing awareness while they learn to be available for themselves.

Transcript: Two-Chair

The client arrived to the session talking about an anxiety pattern where they feel a sense of panic that can only be soothed in connection with others. There doesn't seem to be a reason for the panic, but their thinking tells them that the anxiety is "right" and it needs to stay.

THERAPIST: I see your hands come together like this (shows two fists at the heart like the client just expressed). What do you notice there?

CLIENT: Yeah, I notice a lot of self-protection.

THERAPIST: A lot of self-protection ... I want to invite you to slow down and notice the way your body is holding this. (Silence as client turns towards self-protection) I heard you say that the anxiety predates you, and when the panic comes you can't self-regulate and all the tools you have don't seem to work. (Silence) And I notice your hands have moved to prayer. What do you notice?

CLIENT: I'm in contact with myself. And I can see how my anxiety wants to pull me to some imagined future.

THERAPIST: Are you open to trying something?

CLIENT: Yes.

THERAPIST: I'm wanting to support you in getting some space from the anxiety. Not to make it go away but to be with it more consciously. What do you notice as you say that?

CLIENT: Much more aligned. The yes is a full yes.

THERAPIST: If you were going to name your anxiety, what would you call it?

CLIENT: Anxious Jane.

THERAPIST: Ok. So, if you're willing, I want to invite you to take your hands like this (shows moving energy to other chair) and to take Anxious Jane and put her over there. As you do this, say aloud what you're putting over there, "I'm putting the part of me that ...."

CLIENT: (Uses hands to put Anxious Jane in the chair) I'm putting the part of me that worries and prepares for bad things in this chair. I'm putting the part of me that uses anxiety to feel in control in this chair.

THERAPIST: Yes, and keep taking all of it from your whole body, it might be in your head and your arms ... all of it and just keep putting all of it over there. (Therapist demos. Client keeps eyes closed and gets even more anxiety in the other chair) Yes, and breathe as you get every last bit.

CLIENT: Ok. That's all of it.

THERAPIST: Great. Now just take a few breaths and notice what it's like to get space from Anxious Jane. What do you notice?

CLIENT: Feeling of more spaciousness in my body.

THERAPIST: What would you name the seat you're currently in? If Anxious Jane is over there, who is here?

CLIENT: Um … The only thing that's coming to me is Resistance.

THERAPIST: Okay. So Anxious Jane is there, and Resistance is here. (This clarified the polarity)

CLIENT: Yes.

THERAPIST: Take a few more breaths into the spaciousness. As you see Anxious Jane, how does she seem from this chair? What does her energy look like to you?

CLIENT: Buzzy and I'm wondering how far away I can get because I'm wanting more space. A little ethereal, like not grounded. Shaky energy and a sense of wringing hands and entirely worry and not wanting to not be worried. She wants to convince everyone that she's right to be worried.

THERAPIST: What do you notice when you say that?

CLIENT: Sad. I feel sad because I can't contact her from this chair and I don't want to convince her to feel differently then she feels and yet I do want to convince her to feel differently.

THERAPIST: Say that directly to her.

CLIENT: I don't want to convince you to feel differently than you feel, and I do want to convince you to feel differently than you feel.

THERAPIST: What do you notice?

CLIENT: Sad because I feel like I'm fighting her. Resisting.

THERAPIST: What do you notice in your body?

CLIENT: Frustration. I don't even want to look at her. I want to be here without her.

THERAPIST: Say it directly to her, "I don't want to look at you, it's too much."

CLIENT: (Tears)

THERAPIST: Let the wave come. (Breathes audibly a few times)

CLIENT: I can't say it to her. There's something so resistant. I feel so harsh towards her and I don't want to be harsh.

THERAPIST: It sounds like there's something truer here, "I want to turn away and I want to find compassion for you."

CLIENT: I can see this is how people feel towards me, and this is how I feel about a lot of people. And it feels true. "I want to have compassion for you and I want to turn away because it feels like too much."

THERAPIST: Is there anything else you want to say to her?

CLIENT: I know you are trying to keep me safe, but this isn't what keeps me safe.

THERAPIST: What do you notice in your heart right now?

CLIENT: Openness and compassion for her and for me. A stillness.

THERAPIST: In a moment I am going to ask you to switch chairs, but first I'm wondering how is that for you to hear?

CLIENT: Fine (laughs). Yeah, I feel … I know it's necessary but it's so much better on this side. But I feel willing.

THERAPIST: Ok, so when you're ready, slowly move over to the other seat. Take a minute to check in with your body and notice what you feel like in this chair. (Silence) What do you notice?

CLIENT: (Breath and tears) A sense of isolation. Fear. Wanting to curl up in the fetal position.

THERAPIST: Isolation and despair and wanting to curl up. Stay with your breath and sense the way your body is holding this. (Breath) And to her, in the chair across from you, what would you say to her?

CLIENT: You're not getting it. I'm so scared. You don't see me. You're not listening. I don't feel safe.

THERAPIST: What do you notice in your body as you say that?

CLIENT: Rigidity, anger. My jaw is tight. I'm alone and I don't want to be alone. I'm right and I want people to acknowledge that I'm right.

THERAPIST: What do you notice when you say that?

CLIENT: Less collapsed and more fiery.

THERAPIST: Notice that both are here. "I'm right. I'm going to keep you out, and I'm alone and I want you to validate me." Is there anything you need from her, in the other chair?

CLIENT: To acknowledge that I might be right.

THERAPIST: What do you notice when you say that?

CLIENT: Relaxed. I need this so badly. Just say, "Maybe I'm right."

Soon after, I had the client move to the other chair, and they moved back and forth in collaborative conversation, making room for everything that arose. Remembering there's no right answer; it's all trial and error. The client increased awareness and arrived at self-compassion and eventually liked Anxious Jane once she accessed her power.

Lessons from the Therapy Room

The way the body expresses a person's mental state has always been a fascination of mine. The metaphysical study of the interconnectedness between physical symptoms and mental rigidity is something that I dedicate much of my time to learning. With clients, the physical symptoms are expressed as they talk and offer an entry point into deep transformation.

The first time I explored the somatic integration experiment with a client, I had been watching the way their body changed as they spoke about their polarity. They became heavy and collapsed when talking about their sexual dissatisfaction, and they became animated and excited when talking about what they wanted with their partner. From my zoomed-out perspective, I reflected this to them: "I notice that you seem heavy when you talk about your dissatisfaction, and you seem more excited when you talk about what you want."

When the client affirmed that this resonated with their experience of themselves, I asked if they wanted to try something. Once they agreed, we gained clarity on the polarity that was present: "I'm hearing this as, 'I want you to want me, and go away.'" The client laughed nervously when their inner conflict was distilled down in such a way. "Yep, that's basically it. I want him to want me, but I get so annoyed and feel so awkward that I just want him to go away."

I directed the client to move into "I want you to want me," first, and to express that with their body. Their arms were in a pulling toward movement as they exaggerated this desire to be wanted. After a few minutes, I directed them to move into "Go away." The client showed me with their words and their body their annoyance and hopelessness, with a desire to be alone and hide.

As the client moved through the polarity, they began to see that all of this was theirs, the desire and awkwardness, the longing and hopelessness. Eventually, they found their way into their midline and said, "From here, I want to explore and find a new way." They sat up straight and took a deep breath, and then I directed them to say it again.

Sitting with clients as they find their way through an inner conflict is a deep honor. I did very little in this session, as my client worked through their own struggle. Remembering that this is their work to do, my client accessed their own awareness and wisdom within an otherwise despairing quandary.

Exercise: Move Through a Polarity

Building on the exercise in Chapter 6, use the polarity you identified for this exercise.

Experiencing the somatic integration is a profound way to regulate the nervous system and discover authentic alignment. Either by yourself or guiding another, identify a polarity and find the corresponding shapes in your body.

Take the shape of the most contracted side of the pole and speak from it. Feel that in your body and take a few breaths.

Next, take the opposite shape and speak from it. Exaggerate the shape as you speak.

Then, go back to the contracted shape and speak from it, and then back to the more powerful shape and speak from it.

Move quickly, and then slowly. Eventually, find the midpoint where you are aligned. Find this shape and discover the words.

References

Foschi, R., & Lombardo, G. P. (2006). Lewinian contribution to the study of personality as the alternative to the mainstream of personality psychology in the 20th Century. In J. Trempata et al. (Eds.), *Lewinian psychology. Proceedings of the international conference Kurt Lewin: Contribution to contemporary psychology* (pp. 86–98). Kazimierz Wielky University Press.

Heller, L., & LaPierre, A. (2012). *Healing developmental trauma: How early trauma affects self-regulation, self-image, and the capacity for relationships.* North Atlantic Books.

Lewin, K. (1935). *A dynamic theory of personality.* McGraw-Hill.

Lindorfer, B. (2020). Personality theory in gestalt theoretical psychotherapy: Kurt Lewin's field theory and his theory of systems in tension revisited. *Gestalt Theory, 43*(1): 29–46.

Siegel, D. (2010). *Mindsight: The new science of personal transformation* (Reprint ed.). Bantam.

Chapter 12

Working with an Unfinished Situation

In order to make sense of ourselves and the environment, we unconsciously look for *wholes* to signify completion of the cycle of our experience, known as a gestalt (Clarkson & Caviccia, 2013). A whole cycle of experience begins with a sensation; we then become aware of an emerging need; we mobilize to get that need met; we take action; we contact the environment to get that need; we experience satisfaction; and we withdraw to rest. When each phase in the cycle is successfully contacted, the experience is complete, and a gestalt is formed. As described in Chapter 7 with the *Cycle of Disrupted Contact*, when the environment is unable to meet our need for contact, the contact boundary is disrupted, and the experience lives within us as an unfinished situation, causing us to see ourselves and the environment through the lens of an incomplete gestalt (Perls et al., 1951).

Unmet needs, also known as lack of contact, from one's caregivers during formative moments of development live within the psyche as an unfinished situation. The dissatisfaction of an incomplete experience with a significant person in their life can cause a client to make meaning about themselves and the world based on the lack of contact. Unfinished situations from the past that were particularly stressful or traumatizing remain present now in the form of unexpressed feelings and thoughts (O'Leary & Nieuwstraten, 2001). From this perspective, it may seem to the client that their current distress is being caused by a deficiency in the environment (i.e. a deficiency in other people). While the current environment may be lacking, when the experience of *now* is filtered through the past, the present moment appears more stressful, with fewer opportunities for resolution.

Because the whole of their experience was never completed, the client may think that they will never experience wholeness or completion. At the time of the original incomplete event, they could not effectively get their need for contact met, so they look at the present moment (which lacks contact) as more evidence that the environment will never meet their need. An unfinished situation can be a drain on our clients' energy, especially when they do not realize that these incomplete experiences from the past are influencing how they perceive and interact with the present (O'Leary, 2013). Since past experience cannot be changed, the repair occurs internally in the way a client contacts themselves, making it possible for them to come into presence and contact with the environment.

DOI: 10.4324/9781003521969-15

The Attachment System

The idea that relationships are essential for human development is reinforced through attachment theory. Attachment theory is the study of the emotional bond between a child and their caregiver, showing us how the whole situation in which a child exists contributes to their developing sense of self (Sternek, 2007). Understanding how early childhood attachment bonds impact a client's identity and relationships helps us to understand how their experience of the here and now is influenced by unfinished business (Burley & Freier, 2004).

The attachment system is housed in the nervous system, as the vagus nerve is responsible for a person's social engagement system. When a person feels connected and in contact with the people in their life, their ventral vagal system accesses a sense of calm, and their breathing and heart rate slow down (Porges, 2023). When a person feels disconnected and contact with others is broken, they feel anxious, defensive, or shut down. Emphasizing the "importance of interaction and relationship on development and psychic health or its failure to develop," attachment theory has identified four attachment styles, all of which have different strategies for regulation (Ainsworth et al., 1978):

1. The *anxious attachment style* craves connection and attempts to externally regulate on other people. This attachment style is created with inconsistent caregivers, so the individual wants to know that closeness won't be compromised.
2. The *avoidant attachment style* craves space and internally regulates in solitude. This attachment style is created with caregivers who are neglectful, and the person adapts by closing off to connection.
3. The *disorganized attachment style* craves closeness and space and can switch rapidly between the two. This attachment style is created in the presence of trauma, and the person adapts by trying to find regulation with others, on their own, and often with substances or other addictions. They may also come across as secure and then suddenly switch.
4. The *secure attachment style* is a co-regulating presence with clear and healthy boundaries. This attachment style is created with caregivers who are a consistent presence of attuned safety and clear boundaries.

When a person's attachment wound is stimulated and their nervous system is activated, the mind can have a challenging time distinguishing the past from the present. Dysregulation overrides a person's access to higher consciousness, and they are effectively identified with their attachment wounds, where an emotional injury from the past guides the thinking of their thought-based reality now. Attempting to complete the unfinished situation, the attachment system longs to be met with resonance. This means that the degree to which a person wants emotional closeness is the degree to which the attachment system wants to be met with closeness. Similarly, the degree to which a person wants emotional space is the degree to which the attachment system wants to be met with space.

When we work with an unfinished situation from early childhood, we are likely working with the client's attachment wound. The inner experience of how the client made meaning of themselves and their environment as a result of having their needs unmet becomes the focus. Instead of looking outside of themselves for the solution to their incomplete situation, we support them in looking within and becoming a secure base for themselves, where they give themselves what their environment failed to give them in the past.

For the client who has an anxious attachment style, learning to be a consistent presence within themselves is extremely healing and offers space for a deep inner repair. For the client with an avoidant attachment system, self-compassion and self-love lead them into deeper self-trust, which allows them to open to real connection. For the client with a disorganized attachment, staying in contact with themselves as they vacillate between being okay, being numb, and being anxious helps them to find their way home to themselves.

Spiritual Timeline

When clients think about unfinished situations, their mind looks back to the time when the event took place, which is known as *linear time*. Linear time is the same as clock time, where clients relate to events according to the past, present, or future. They may try to remember a specific event that caused their attachment injury and the age they were when it took place. While this may be useful to the client, looking back in time takes them out of presence (Figure 12.1).

Working in the present moment with something that happened in the past requires that clients access *spiritual time*, which is nonlinear time of spiritual dimensions. Opening to awake awareness, clients are able to access the consciousness of the imprint of the incomplete experience. Instead of thinking back to a memory, they bring their attention to the energetic quality of the young one who still exists within them. In the present moment, clients relate to their inner young one in the experience they had that was unfinished. They may also relate to future versions of themselves and who they are becoming (Figure 12.2).

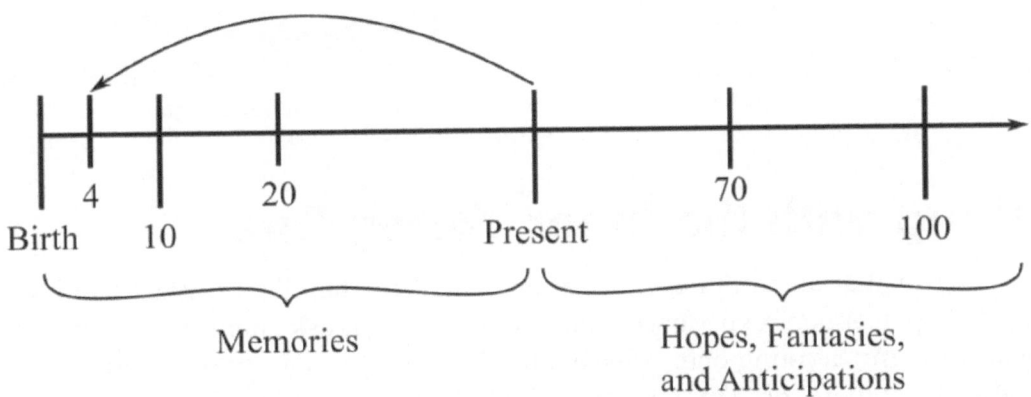

Figure 12.1 Linear Time

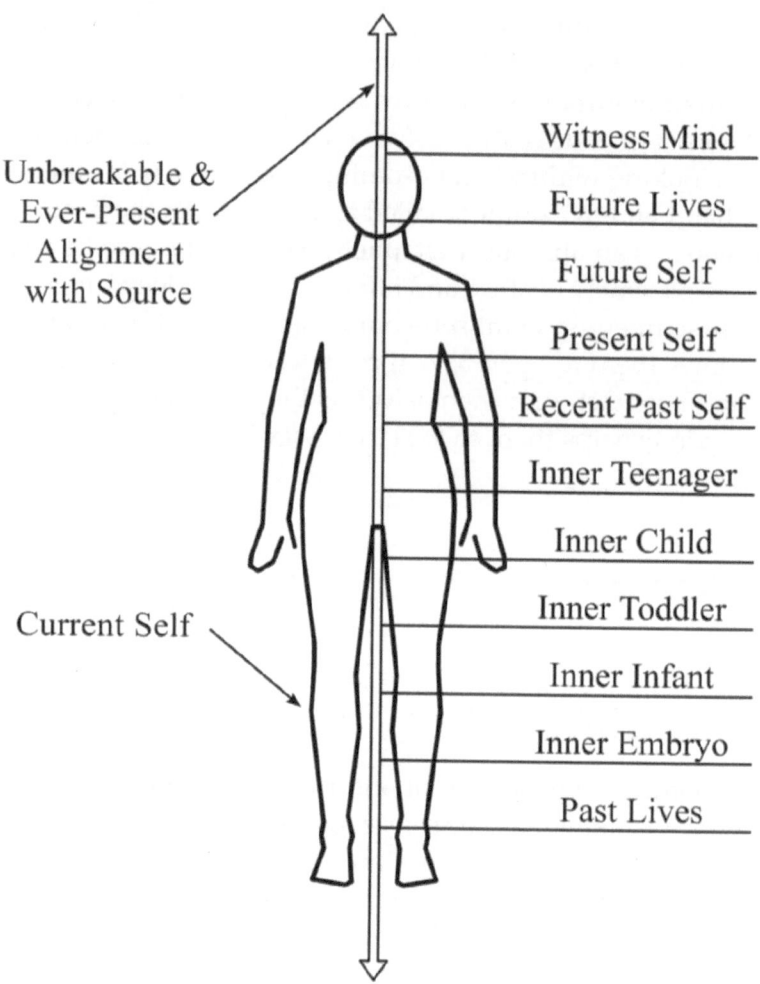

Figure 12.2 Spiritual Time (Kwiker, 2023, p. 136)

When we shift the relationship to time, what happened in the past is accessible now. Time is such a huge component of how people relate to the world, and the spiritual experience of timelessness supports a client's healing potential. Healing happens in the present moment, and through spiritual time, we can access different aspects of a client in the here and now.

Working with the Inner Young One

When we sense that an unfinished situation seated in the client's attachment system is guiding their perception, experience, and actions, we can ask them if they would like to work with their inner young one: "I have attention on a younger part of you. What do you notice when I say that?" or "I'm wondering if you're interested in working with your inner young one?"

If the client is interested in working with their inner young one, either we can invite them to close their eyes and look at their inner young one, or we can invite them to put the young one in a chair or on the sofa next to them. Once the inner young one is explicitly present, we collaboratively work with the client to discover what it is they need in order to complete the unfinished situation.

What follows are guidelines that may be useful to consider as you proceed:

- Ask the client what they notice when they look at their inner young one.
- Invite them to **witness** their younger self, saying to them, "I see you. I see that you feel (powerless, alone, angry, scared, sad, unlovable, etc.)."
- Ask them if there is anything they want to **say** to their young one?
- Ask them if there is anything their inner young one **needs** from them.
- Invite them to wrap them in **love**. The client can say to the young one, "I see you. I see that you feel (scared). I see you and I love you."
- Invite them to **validate** their young one: "It makes sense to me that you feel (powerless, alone, scared, sad, etc.)."
- Invite them to **honor** their young one's wisdom: "You were so wise to (develop this strategy)."
  - Note: If you had the inner young one in a chair, consider having the client sit in the seat of the young one to receive self-love.
- Support them in **clearing the introjection**: *Since the misbelief is acquired, it can be returned.* If the young one/client is ready to stop carrying around this misbelief, invite them to give it back.
- They may need to call on the cosmic realm for support, asking their ancestors, Buddha nature, Universe, or guides to help clear the energy they're holding that does not belong to them.
- If the young one is not ready to give it back, it is likely because they feel responsible. If this is the case, check in to see what they want to tell their young one about the misbelief.
- Ask them to tell their young one **what is true**. Since the misbelief that the inner young one created was false, ask the client if they have anything they want to say to their young one. Example: *"You are safer honoring yourself."*
- Invite them to **commit to the repair**. The client can make a commitment to honor their young one in the way they need: *"I will always honor your power."* Repeating this several times allows the young one to really take it in.
- Next, **update** the inner young one. "I'm (current age) years old." And then, invite the client to take their young one's hand and show them their life now.
  - Note: If a client is not happy with where their life is now, this might be painful. Whatever arises is important for the client to feel as they integrate and update the young one.
- Invite the client to **affirm their truth and anchor repair**. After the young one orients to current time, affirm the truth they just said to their young one from the first person: "I am ready to (*claim my power*)."
- Claiming one's truth is a powerful punctuation at the end of this process. Repeat the statement three times to really anchor it in.

Moving into Power

When a client has built a life based on trying to resolve unfinished business, they likely have unfulfilled hopes and dreams for the future. As a client shares their unfulfilled dreams, we can listen to any insecurities or old stories about themselves that are holding them back. If so inspired, we can ask them if they'd like to do an experiment with their future self, sometimes called the *seat of power*.

Working with their power may help to illuminate any unfinished business and support them in being more clear and present as they move forward on their path. In the spiritual realm of time, their future self already dwells within. Inviting their future self to be present in the session allows the client to work with any blocks they have to owning their power.

As with the inner young one, working with the future self can be done with a two-chair technique, where one chair is the seat of power, and the current chair is the voice of insecurity. Another way to do this is with a visualization, where the client closes their eyes and sees their future self internally. These experiments come to mind when a client really wants to accomplish something but has imposter syndrome or is afraid they will never be enough to manifest their dreams.

What follows are some guidelines to consider with this experiment:

♦   If the client is interested in trying an experiment, set up the context as described in Chapter 10.

♦   Bring in a second chair and name it the seat of power, or some other name that resonates with the client. This is the seat of their future self, and it houses something relevant to who they want to become.

♦   Invite the client to look at the seat of their future self and describe how they seem (i.e. powerful, confident, happy …).

♦   Ask the client what they notice when they see that version of themselves.

♦   Ask them if there is anything they want to say to their future self.

♦   Work with any constructs that are preventing the client from moving into that seat. Shame, insecurities, attachment wounds, anticipatory fear, and so on are explored in depth.

♦   Once the client has deepened awareness and regulated their nervous system, ask them if they are ready to move into the seat of their future self.

♦   Have them experience the phenomenology of their seat of power. Ask them what they notice as they sit here.

♦   Ask them if there is anything this aspect of themselves wants to say.

♦   Perhaps the experiment ends here, or perhaps you continue until they seem complete.

Transcript: Completing Unfinished Business

Client arrived to session talking about their excitement about a new project and then the inner experience of no motivation. Even though this seemed like a polarity that we might work with, it turned out that the client deepened into awareness around an attachment wound related to work ethic and being told they were lazy.

THERAPIST: If your jaw had a voice, what would it say?

CLIENT: I can't let go.

THERAPIST: What do you notice as you say that?

CLIENT: Tears in my eyes and a sweetness and recognition of my inner experience. It's very body-based. "I'm holding so much. I'm working so hard."

THERAPIST: Stay with yourself there. Take a few breaths. What do you notice now?

CLIENT: Release.

THERAPIST: "I'm holding so much. I'm working so hard."

CLIENT: Sadness and tenderness.

THERAPIST: Making room for sadness and tenderness. Let the tears come if they want to come. Staying with yourself, and you can close your eyes if you want. (Client closes eyes) Keep inviting that wave to move through you. (Silence) What do you notice now?

CLIENT: My breath is deepening. And I see that I have a story about myself that I'm not working enough or doing much, but when you reflected those words back to me "I work so hard …" it's like, tiredness makes sense.

THERAPIST: Yes! That makes sense to me. The narrative is different from the embodied experience.

CLIENT: Yes. My mind wants to argue about this, like I don't work so hard.

THERAPIST: Let me hear more from the voice. "It's not true …"

CLIENT: It's not true. You're lazy. (Tears) And I feel a collapse in my shoulders and gut … everything wanting to come forward.

THERAPIST: Close your eyes and notice the way your body holds that. Let it know you see it and you're listening. Does this voice belong to you or did you pick it up somewhere?

CLIENT: It does not belong to me. I would say my mom and grandfather.

THERAPIST: What do you notice when you say that aloud?

CLIENT: Relief that it's not mine. It's external, like what people will think of me if I'm not showing that I'm doing enough. Like other people decide the truth of me. Am I ready to let that go?

THERAPIST: What do you notice when you say that?

CLIENT: More sadness. And I feel really young. (The client's inner young one was present)

THERAPIST: Staying there with the young one. What would you tell your young one about this?

CLIENT: F them! It's not true. What they say about you isn't true.

THERAPIST: What do you notice in your body?

CLIENT: Tension in my jaw. Anger.

THERAPIST: Yes, anger. Feel that anger, and give it a tone with the exhale if you want. (Groans)

CLIENT: (Groans)

THERAPIST: Let's bring all our attention to your young one. I really want her to be seen right now. Looking at her … what do you notice when you see her?

CLIENT: Mad.

THERAPIST: Yeah. Keep seeing her. Seeing that she's mad.

CLIENT: She just wants to scream because they're crazy.

THERAPIST: Keep seeing her for that and validating that anger. (Silence) Yeah. And let's get them completely out of her field. Is that okay? (Yes) See them as they're small, like 1 inch tall. It's not to make them small but to make more room for her. (Silence) Let her see how small they are. What do you notice?

CLIENT: She's safe.

THERAPIST: Feel that in your body, and let her feel that safety. And if there is any part of this misbelief that she's lazy that she wants to give back to them, inviting her to do that. Any part of this that is not part of her true nature and doesn't belong to her … just giving it back. What do you notice?

CLIENT: I see that something just came back into alignment, and I can see that as a Leo it is my true nature to hunt when I want to hunt, and I rest in the sun when it's time to rest. And I feel this sense of power.

THERAPIST: I think I'm hearing this as you know when it's time to work and when it's time to rest.

CLIENT: Yes. I feel the congruence of that.

THERAPIST: Tell your young one that: "You know when it's time to work and when it's time to rest." Is there anything else you'd want to tell her about that?

CLIENT: Yeah, it's a little sticky, but I want to say something about the world. Like … it's an upside-down world with a value on productivity. But I don't know how to resolve that.

THERAPIST: And I see your hands like this (shows a bubble around young one) as you say that.

CLIENT: Yeah, I see us in a bubble.

THERAPIST: Keep using your hands like that to sense into that bubble. (Repeats movement several times) What do you notice?

CLIENT: (Smiles) There's like this mother energy that's holding and loving. And the world is crazy, but I'm here and I'm solid and this is where things are sane.

THERAPIST: What do you notice when you say that? "This is where things are sane."

CLIENT: Yummy. It's so true.

THERAPIST: Say it again. "This is where things are sane."

CLIENT: This is true. This is where things are sane, and I've got you.

After reparenting the inner young one, the client arrived at commitment to her young one to honor her natural rhythm, which turned into the affirmation, "I will always honor my natural rhythm."

Lessons from the Therapy Room

I was sitting with a client who I had been working with for a few years. They arrived to their session talking about how they felt more aligned and connected to themselves than they ever remembered feeling. The health and vitality of their subtle energy body was obvious to my metaphysical eyes, and we were celebrating this experience of moving in the world from a place of honoring themselves rather than betraying themselves as they previously had.

"The one area that I've noticed anxiety is in my dating life," they said.

They had been dating a person who they had strong feelings for, but that person wasn't ready to commit in the way my client wanted. Because of this, my client started dating another person at the same time. This was an ethical decision where all people involved knew that they were not monogamous.

"Each time this new person texts me, my heart drops," they shared.

"Your heart drops."

"Yes, I can feel it right now as I share it with you."

"If your heart had a voice, what would it say?" I asked.

"I'm not sure." The client closed their eyes. "Hmm, I think it's saying 'I'm scared that I'm in trouble.'"

"You're scared that you're in trouble. What do you notice when you say that?"

"I feel confused. I know I'm not in trouble. I know that I'm acting from integrity, but I think [the person I've been dating for a while] will get upset that this other person's texting me. It's strange, though, because I've told [this person] that I'm seeing [this other person]."

"Let's bring our attention to your heart," I invited. "Let your heart know that you see that it's scared of getting in trouble." Some silence and contemplative attention was placed on the client's heart. "As you sit with your heart, I start sensing a younger part of yourself. What do you notice when I say that?"

"Well, I'm emotional," they said while wiping away their tears. "I don't understand why, though."

"That's okay. Let the emotion move through you even if you don't understand why it's here."

"Ugh, I wasn't expecting this. My arms are feeling tingly and I just want to cry."

"As you notice the way your body is holding this, is it okay if we put attention on your inner young one?"

"Yes," they replied. "Oh. I see. I was so afraid of getting in trouble when my step-father sexually abused me. I thought it was my fault."

"Stay with your young one and let them know that you see they're scared and afraid that what's happened is their fault."

"Ugh, I want to scream. It wasn't my fault! Why do I think it was my fault?!"

"Say that to them, 'It wasn't your fault. What happened was not your fault.' What do you notice?"

"My mom's voice. She told me it was my fault in several different ways. And when I finally told the school counselor, my mom blamed me for bringing shame to the family."

"What do you notice when you remember that?"

"I'm so mad at her. This is not my shame. This is his shame."

"Yes, tell your inner young one this truth. You have nothing to be ashamed of. This is not your fault."

"This isn't your shame, it's his. He should be ashamed, not you. He knows he did something wrong. You did nothing wrong. You did the right thing by telling someone about this."

As the client cleared the introjection of mom and step-dad, they gave themselves what they needed. They opened up to themselves even more as they completed this unfinished situation. Because this trauma was so complex, the client may have this wound emerge in other ways at different times. However, they have more access to their wise self to support themselves through the emotional dysregulation.

At the end of the session, the client was buzzing, and their energy body was full. They expressed the clarity they were experiencing in relationship to their life, their mom, and their partners. Their breath was full, and they were present in the here and now. They began to see new possibilities for themselves, and they were contemplating talking with their mom about this situation from the past.

Exercise: Attach to Self

The following sentence stems are powerful invitations to be a secure base for yourself. You can offer them to your clients as homework, and you can use them in your own real-time transformation.

- ♦ When I am emotionally activated, my inner young one needs _____ from me.
- ♦ When I am enacting my habitual pattern of _____, my inner young one needs _____ from me.

References

Ainsworth, M. D. S., Blehar, M. C., Waters, E., & Wall, S. (1978). *Patterns of attachment: A psychological study of the strange situation.* Lawrence Erlbaum.

Burley, T., & Freier, M. (2004). Character Structure: A Gestalt Cognitive Theory. *Psychotherapy Theory Research Practice Training, 41*(3): 321–331.

Clarkson, P., & Caviccia, S. (2013). *Gestalt counseling in action* (4th ed.). Sage Publications Ltd.

Kwiker, H. (2023). *Align: Living and loving from the true self* (pp. 395–411). Mantra Books.

O'Leary, E. (Ed.). (2013). *Gestalt therapy around the world*. Wiley-Blackwell.

O'Leary, E., & Nieuwstraten, I. M. (2001). Unfinished business in gestalt reminiscence therapy: A discourse analytic study. *Counseling Psychology Quarterly, 12*(4): 310–318.

Perls, F., Hefferline, R., & Goodman, P. (1951). *Gestalt therapy: Excitement and growth in the human personality*. London: Souvenir Press.

Porges, S. W. (2023). *Our polyvagal world: How safety and trauma change us*. W. W. Norton & Company.

Sternek, K. (2007). Attachment theory and Gestalt psychology. *Gestalt Theory, 29*(4).

Chapter 13

Working with Different Contact Boundary Disturbances

When we work with a client's contact boundary disturbances, we are working with the adaptive strategies they created to break contact during moments when the environment was unable to meet their needs. Where these adaptive strategies were once a way to get relief from the dysfunction of the environment, they have become rigid ways of being that cause the client distress. When the boundary between the client and their environment is unclear, there is a disturbance of contact and awareness (Perls, 1973). *Distinguishing* themselves from others, and *connecting* with themselves and others, are functions of a boundary.

Awake awareness allows a client to perceive a situation accurately, which leads to self-responsibility. Self-responsibility is the *ability* to *respond* to one's inner and outer experience from their True *Self*. This is *not* synonymous with hyper-independence. When a client is aware and in full contact, they know *what* they do, *how* they do it, that they have alternatives, and that they are *choosing* to be as they are. A client "who verbally acknowledges [their] situation but does not really see it, *know* it, *react* to it and *feel* in response to it is not fully aware and is not in full contact" (Yontef, 1993).

Any narrative that a client shares is an opportunity to explore how their mind is disrupting contact, where there is no distinction between themselves and others (Perls, 1973). As we listen to their words, we can follow the thread of their thought back to the client, discovering what unfinished business lives beneath this thought pattern. Instead of being induced into their disrupted contact, we must cultivate the skill of witnessing their patterns and meeting them at the contact boundary. When we are able to see the whole configuration clearly, we can create openings for the client to work with their contact boundary disruptions.

Discovering one's own boundaries requires effective self-regulation, making it possible to be aware of potentially *nourishing* or *toxic* elements in the environment. Self-trust is essential to meeting the environment at the contact boundary, and this is cultivated through honoring their somatic sensations, intuition, needs, and desires. Bringing a quality of inner security with them as they contact the environment allows what is nourishing to be integrated, and what is toxic is rejected (Yontef, 1993).

Once a client is able to make contact at the boundary point, they quickly learn the difference between "ideas and ideation, between well-worn obsessional pathways and new thoughts, between a statement of experience and a statement of a statement" (Yontef, 1993). Because the client's awareness, experience, and insight are the essence of this work, they are offered the opportunity to make these distinctions on their own accord. This, of course, empowers them to bring this awareness and ability with them into all facets of life.

DOI: 10.4324/9781003521969-16

Working with Deflections

Deflection is the way a client avoids contact by turning away from uncomfortable emotions. The act of turning away avoids the discomfort of expressing directly, in an effort to be polite (Yontef, 1993). It also prevents them from being affected by the environment, allowing them to be untouched by the world around them. Deflections can be expressed through looking away from a person, talking incessantly, being vague, minimizing their own and others' experience, and talking *about* themselves (Polster & Polster, 1973).

At the moment when the strategy of deflection was first developed, a client was wise to disrupt contact. Turning away offered a sense of differentiation from the environment when they otherwise were dependent on those around them. Without the inner resources or relational support to regulate their nervous system, deflecting was an attempt at finding inner balance.

With the relational support of the therapist, a client can become aware of the way they deflect. Increased awareness combined with direct contact with the therapist offers them a space to explore turning toward themselves. As they stay with the discomfort of their emotional experience, they begin to move through unfinished business and find their way back home to themselves.

Mapping out the way a client turns away from themselves with great compassion allows the therapeutic field to be a place for the client to return to contact with themselves.

Here are some ways to support increasing awareness with deflections:

♦ "I see you looking over there. I want to invite you to notice how you feel as you turn away."
♦ "It seems like you just turned away from yourself. What do you notice?"
♦ "As you were talking about sadness, I noticed you laughed. What do you notice in your body?"
♦ "It seems like you just left yourself. Where are you right now?"
♦ "It seems like there's a lot happening in your body right now. What do you notice?"
♦ "You said that you're feeling a lot … then you started talking about your partner … what do you notice on the level of sensation in your body?"
♦ "I heard you say you feel numb. Tell me more about numbness."
♦ "You said that you *understand* why this is happening. I'm curious how you *feel* in relationship to this event?"

Examples of working with deflection:

♦ Invite the client to close their eyes and sense into the body. "What do you notice with your eyes closed?"
♦ Invite the client to explore turning away consciously. They can look away while you look away, too. You can explore contact while turning away. "What happens in the body while consciously turning away?"

- ◆ Experiment with distance. The client or the therapist can move further away and use this movement to increase awareness. "What happens in the body when we move further away?"
- ◆ Invite the client to move their body, such as to shake their arms or get up and move, to discharge the discomfort. "What do you notice now that you've moved?"
- ◆ Invite the client to allow their emotions to move through them. Any place you see bracing or turning away, invite more awareness to that place. For example, "Opening your throat and allowing that wave [of emotion] to move through you."
- ◆ Bring awareness to where the energy is concentrated. If the client is talking *about* themselves, you may say, "It seems like there's a lot of energy up here (pointing to the mind). What do you notice up here?"

Remember, we don't want to change clients. We simply want to bring more awareness to their patterns to support their increasing awareness. To meet our client where they are, we must stay in contact with them as they leave contact. When we invite them to attend to themselves while turning away, we begin to interrupt their patterns of disconnection. By tending to the ways they disconnect from themselves, we're essentially teaching them how to regulate their nervous system and reminding their whole system that they are now safe to be in contact.

When we are in contact with our Self, the place where a deflection previously lived now holds our inherent connection with our Self. Through this connection, we are able to honor the wisdom of our body's sensations.

Working with Introjections

Introjections are internalized beliefs, feelings, and ways of being that are taken in whole without contemplating their truth or resonance with our true nature. Absorbing environmental material without assimilating or discriminating causes a client to create a personality based on the presumption that the environment was healthy and the reflection from others was accurate (Perls, 1973). This leads to rigid characteristics, where the client is attempting to fit into the values they introjected, imposing them on themselves.

Taking in environmental material was, in a sense, a way to find belonging. By believing what others told them about themselves and about the world, a client gained a sense of connection. However, introjections disrupt contact by way of conforming to the environment without discrimination. Introjections commonly present as a delusion or misbelief, the voice of *should*, and shame-based thoughts (i.e. beliefs that they are unlovable, that they are responsible for other people, etc.).

Because introjections were acquired at a time when a client did not have a sense of self separate from the environment, they may not identify these ideas as something that was acquired. As a personality characteristic that has been with them for a long time, they seem, to the client, a part of who they are. Any belief that causes a client distress and seems to deviate from their true nature is likely an introjection. With our reflection and curiosity, clients can discover where they acquired these ideas, who they belong to, and what is actually true about themselves.

Listening for themes of beliefs, emotions, and patterned ways of being, we can discover the introjection that is embedded in their words. Reflecting the deeper essence of what they're saying, we can then ask them how they relate to that belief.

Here are some ways to help a client identify an introjection:

♦ "I hear you saying that (you're too emotional). I'm wondering when you started thinking that about yourself?" This gives the client an opportunity to identify when they acquired this introjection.

♦ "It sounds like you believe (that you're too much for other people). What do you notice as you contemplate that belief?" This gives the client the opportunity to consider times in their early life when their caregivers couldn't meet their needs.

♦ "I heard you say that you (feel responsible for the people in your life). What is underneath this belief?" This gives the client an opportunity to look deeper within themselves to discover why they think what they think.

♦ "When you say that you (need to set better boundaries), I hear that as 'I am (accustomed to betraying myself).' What do you notice when I say that?" This gives the client an opportunity to see the way they manipulate the environment, which leads to deeper curiosity about where they acquired the belief that connection occurs through self-betrayal.

♦ "It sounds like you (think you should be more driven at work). Is that voice yours?" This gives them an opportunity to discover if this is what they think or if they have picked this idea up somewhere.

♦ "I have attention on the voice of 'Not good enough.' I'm wondering who that voice belongs to?" This is useful in differentiating from the introjection, especially when the therapist is clear that the misbelief has been acquired.

Once an introjection is identified as such, we can support the client in increasing awareness in relationship to the belief. This helps a client to unblend from these acquired ideas and values, digest what they want to take in, and give back what is not in alignment with the truth of who they are. Some ways to experiment with clearing introjections include:

♦ Invite the client to close their eyes and see the "voice of" the introjection as if it's sitting in front of them. They may spontaneously say, "That's the voice of my [caregiver]!" Give the client space to talk about what was happening in their life when they took in this idea. Work to repair the unfinished business, where the client has the opportunity to give themselves what they needed then. This supports them in completing the gestalt and building self-trust.

♦ Invite the client to put the introjection in a chair. Direct the client to use their body to move the energy of this voice to the other chair. Let them know that you are not trying to get rid of it, but that you want to learn from it. Ask them, "What do you notice when you get space from this voice?" Clients may spontaneously see this as the voice of their caregiver, sibling, teacher, or some other primary attachment figure in their childhood.

♦ If the client has identified that the voice does not belong to them, you can ask them what they want to say to it, what they want to do with it, and/or what is actually true about themselves. This invitation has no right or wrong answer. It is the exploration itself that disrupts homeostasis.

♦ You can invite the client to transmute the voice or give it back, according to what they say they want. You can invite the client to use their awareness and breath to clear any beliefs that do not originate with them. You can also make space for them to invite in spirit guides, helpers, fairies, and so on to help clear anything that is not theirs to process.

♦ It may emerge that this is an inter-generational pattern, and you can invite the client to see the pattern in their lineage. If that resonates with the client, you can invite them to sense into their ancestors. Looking all the way back to where the misbelief was first created, they can call on their ancestors for support to undo this pattern. Next, you can invite them to see the younger generation in front of them, noticing how the pattern is transforming now, in real time.

When we are in contact with our Self, the place where an introjection previously lived now holds our ability to know what we value and what we believe to be true, as well as our ability to be curious about another person's truth.

Working with Projections

When a person does not take responsibility for their own inner state and actions, and instead they assign blame to their environment, they are projecting (Naranjo, 2004). "Projection is a confusion of self and other that results from attributing to the outside something that is truly self" (Yontef, 1993). Being unaware of what originates within one's self leads the person to infer that the outside world is at fault for how they feel within.

Projections can have both a negative and a positive expression, where a person assigns responsibility for both positive and negative experiences to their environment. An example of a negative projection is when a client is talking about an ex-partner who treated them poorly. Upon further reflection, the client realizes that they had moments of intuition during the relationship that they ignored. Ignoring their own intuition is the way they treated themselves poorly, and they are assigning their pattern of self-betrayal to their ex-partner.

An example of a positive projection is when a client is in a new relationship and they talk about how excited they are that this person is so amazing. They are assigning their positive feelings to the other person, causing them to make the other person the source of their happiness. When disappointment occurs, this positive projection can quickly turn negative, where the other person becomes the source of their frustration and anger. Without taking responsibility for their own emotions, the relationship becomes an illusion of their projections rather than deep contact.

When a client is talking about someone in a negative light, there is something negative in their own shadow that they are not in touch with. When a client is talking about someone in a positive light, there is something positive in their shadow that they are denying. Owning their experience and taking responsibility for their blind spots is what allows a client to make contact at the boundary.

During a session with an individual client, we can hear their projections through the narratives they have about other people. The meaning they make of other people's behavior is an indicator of something deeper within the client's shadow. Projections often sound like blame and resentment, especially when they do not give voice to their own contribution to the dynamic. Projections can also present as the client believing other people have the power. Similarly, when asked what they want, a client who makes projections wants other people to be different.

When a client is talking about a person who is not in the room currently, we can follow that thread back to the client to discover who they are in this dynamic. What the client says about the other person gives us insight into the client themselves.

Here are some ways to bring attention to a projection:

♦ "As you talk about [this person], what do you notice in your body?"
♦ "It seems like a lot of your attention is on [this other person]."
♦ "As you share your story about [this person], what do you notice about yourself?"
♦ "You said you were angry. Let me hear from the voice of anger." After the client vents from anger, ask them, "What do you notice as you say that?" To bring the attention back to the client, ask them, "What does anger need right now?"
♦ "It seems like [this person] is mirroring something for you. What do you notice with their reflection?"
♦ "As you talk about [this person], it seems like they have a lot of power over your state of being. What are you noticing?"
♦ "I heard you say that they [have been unsupportive]. I also heard you say that you [don't want to support them]. What do you notice when I reflect that?"

Projection can be seen in a clinical setting when a client talks about a person in their lives, but it can also be seen by the way the client treats the clinician. When the client is projecting onto the clinician, there is a profound opportunity to access the projection in real time:

♦ "You seem to place a lot of your attention on me. What are you noticing?"
♦ "It seems like you're shining all your light on me. What do you notice about you?"
♦ "When you ask me what I think, I wonder what's happening for you there."
♦ "When you say you wish you could bring me with you, I'm wondering what's beneath that for you."

Here are examples of working with projections:

♦ Mapping out the relational dynamic as a clear mirror, without getting hooked into the client's narrative, is extremely powerful to increase the client's awareness.
♦ Because projections involve perceptions of other people, it can be useful to begin by inviting the client to energetically get the other person out of the room. You can say to them, "If it's okay with you, I'd like to invite you to get [this person] out of the room. Let them be where they are." This can increase awareness immensely, in and

of itself. Then, inviting the client to take a few breaths and feel into having more space for themselves.

♦ Once the other person is out of the room, you have space to work with the client's inner-subjective experience. Many times, an attachment wound is activated in the dynamic with the other person, so this can be a good time to resolve unfinished business.

♦ When the client has deepened into contact with themselves, you can then presence the other person. In doing so, you are discovering how they relate to this person now that they have worked to repair their attachment system. This is called an *empty chair experiment*, and it is best done after a client has cleared the projection. "If they were here right now, what would you say to them?" It can be helpful to let the client know that you want their uncensored truth, and that this isn't something you're asking them to go say to the other person.

When we are in contact with our Self, the place where a projection previously lived now holds our capacity for intuitive clarity and empathic curiosity.

Working with Retroflections

Retroflections are how a person treats themselves in the way they want to treat someone else, substituting self for environment (Yontef, 1993). This internal movement of *turning in on one's self* had an adaptive quality when the environment was not welcoming of the person's authentic expression. For example, holding in their anger toward their caregivers when it wasn't safe to express was a wise way to find homeostasis. This provided an illusion of self-sufficiency, where the person could disrupt contact with the environment by containing their anger within themselves.

When a client is antagonistic with themselves, has a strong inner critic, or has perfectionistic tendencies, these indicate a possible retroflection. As long as the energy of the retroflection is being turned in on oneself, the natural flow of energy is thwarted. A person cannot find their way out of a retroflection without directing that energy where it originally needed to go while in the safety of a clinical setting.

Here are some ways to conceptualize working with retroflections:

♦ Authentic expression in the right direction moves the energy of the retroflection.

♦ Since a retroflection is a turning on oneself, one option is to put the caregiver in a chair and have them say to the caregiver what their inner critic has turned inward.

♦ Another option is to put the inner critic in the chair and discover what it is polarized against. Then, proceed with two-chair. As you work with this, you may touch on introjected ideas that need to be cleared.

Because retroflections may be hard to identify, here is an example that may help to clarify this concept:

> CLIENT: "I'm such a redneck hillbilly. When am I going to grow up and get it together?"
>
> THERAPIST: "When I hear these words, I imagine your young one wanted to say this to your dad. 'You're a redneck hillbilly, dad. When are you going to grow up and get it together?' What do you notice when I say that?"
>
> CLIENT: (Through tears) "Oh my goodness. Absolutely. If I was safe enough to say that, I would have said that to him."
>
> THERAPIST: "What do you notice in your body right now?"
>
> CLIENT: "I feel like I'm a real person, like I have form and depth. I feel so seen right now."
>
> THERAPIST: "Are you open to trying something with this?"
>
> CLIENT: "Yes."
>
> THERAPIST: "Imagine your dad was in the chair over there, and say those words to him. What do you notice when I suggest that?"
>
> CLIENT: "I feel a little scared, like I'm going to upset him and I'll see his rage."
>
> THERAPIST: "Notice that there's fear here, and let's make room for fear. (Silence. Breath) I want to remind you that I'm not suggesting that you actually say this to him. Here, in the safety of this container, I want to make room for your full truth to have space."
>
> CLIENT: "Yeah, I want that too. I need a minute. (Silence) Dad, when are you going to grow up and be an adult?"
>
> THERAPIST: "What do you notice when you say that?"
>
> CLIENT: "I feel a surge of energy, like, yeah, I want to know! When are you going to grow up?"

When we are in contact with our Self, the place where a retroflection previously lived now holds our capacity to speak our sovereign truth.

Working with Confluence

Alternating between connecting and separating is the function of a healthy boundary. In unhealthy states, a boundary vacillates between merging with others and being inaccessible to others. When a person merges with their environment, their state of confluence blurs the distinction between self and other, and the boundary is lost (Yontef, 1998). When a person is inaccessible to the environment, a person isolates and loses awareness of the importance of others.

In infancy, caregivers are responsible for providing healthy boundaries. Because a baby is born in a state of confluence, a growing child needs help from their caregivers to learn safe and healthy contact. *Merging with* the environment is an attempt at holding onto an experience or perceived contact when healthy contact is not provided. *Isolating from* the environment is an attempt at not needing others when healthy contact is not provided.

When we attune to the client's energetic expression, their boundary appears dispersed. Diminishing one's boundaries also diminishes one's self. A client who is in confluence has a challenge with knowing what they want, making it hard for them to ask for what they want and saying "no" to the requests of others. Because their sense of well-being is tied up in the well-being of others, they often process other people's emotions. They lack access to their own sense of self, and they often feel confused as to what they think and feel.

Here are some ways to work with confluence:

♦ It is helpful to energetically get other people out of the room so you can see the client when they are not merged with others. As you do this, give plenty of time and silence for them to notice how they feel. Invite them to use their breath and awareness to take up more space energetically.

♦ If the client has a hard time letting go of other people's energy, invite them to imagine the other person as 1 inch tall. Affirm for them that this is not to make the other person small, but instead, it is to make more room for themselves. This shift in perspective is powerful in supporting clients in differentiating from the environment.

♦ If the client still has a hard time letting go of other people's emotions, invite them to put them into a vessel, like a crystal pyramid. This is especially helpful if there is trauma involved.

♦ Once they have a separate sense of self, support them in creating energetic boundaries. (This is described in Chapter 7: Creating Healthy Boundaries exercise.)

♦ When they have adequate inner support and clear boundaries, you can offer the vagal toning experiment, where they practice saying "No" as you role play as a person in their life. (This is described in Chapter 6: Exercises for Safety and Connection.)

♦ After boundaries are set, invite other people's energy back into the room while directing the client to stay in contact with themselves. Ask the client what they notice in their body. Ask the client if the other people believe that they are separate.

♦ If the client's eyes have been closed, once the contact boundary is set, invite them to slowly open their eyes. As they do this, instruct them to stay in contact with themselves and to breathe as they titrate to opening their eyes. Eventually, have them look into your eyes. If they lose contact with themselves, they can close their eyes again. This is a practice of contacting themselves while contacting the environment.

When we are in contact with our Self, the place where confluence previously lived now holds our capacity to meet others at the contact boundary while experiencing the spiritual oneness of our interconnection with all of life.

Lessons from the Therapy Room

Working with couples offers a potent container to see the way contact boundary disturbances interrupt connection in real time. I recall a time when I was working with a couple who had been married for ten years. They owned a business together, and all of their recreational activities were done together. Although they spent the majority of their time together, they argued daily about work, sex, and money.

One spouse (we will call them Erin) demonstrated a high degree of perfectionistic and anxious characteristics, and they were in charge of organizing finances, marketing, and other logistics. The other spouse (we will call them Ryan) demonstrated procrastination and avoidant characteristics, and they were in charge of the people and product side of the business. Erin displayed characteristics of an insecure attachment style, and Ryan displayed characteristics of an avoidant attachment style.

Erin wanted things done in a certain way and at a certain time. Ryan would agree to these requests and then consistently not follow through. Both the people in the couple appeared to be extremely angry with one another and unable to self-regulate. Erin was expressive with their blame, and they wanted Ryan to change so they could feel better. Ryan was more passive-aggressive with their resentment, trying to give Erin what they wanted to get them to calm down.

Each time they arrived at the session, Erin came with a litany of offenses that they were holding against Ryan. Ryan would come with a desire to find a way to stop the conflict, along with a lot of confusion and defensiveness. The nervous system of the couple was continuously overcome with fight or flight. Ryan didn't feel safe because they sensed Erin's judgment, and Erin didn't feel safe because they sensed Ryan's incongruence.

Because Erin often raised their voice and was unable to regulate, much of the early work was focused on co-regulating with both of them so they felt heard and could be present with one another. Similarly, because Ryan appeared passive-aggressive and would agree to things they were not following through with, the earlier work for them focused on getting to an inner place of congruence.

When working with couples, the internal polarities are externalized in the room through one another's reflection. In this instance, Erin was anxious for connection, while Ryan was avoidant. Erin was perfectionistic, while Ryan let things go. Erin asked for what they wanted, while Ryan disowned their desire. It's easy to see here that what one person disowned, the other embodied, and vice versa. When each person has the opportunity to integrate their shadow and complete unfinished business, they can meet at the contact boundary and have true connection.

Over the course of our work together, Erin was able to increase awareness of the way they turned away from their emotions and projected them onto Ryan. They worked with an introjection acquired in infancy, where they were left to cry it out in their crib, and the family story was that their emotions were too much for everyone. Erin could see that their emotions were too much for themselves because they had never learned how to stay with their experience. They could also see that they merged with Ryan through sex in order to have a sense of connection, which set up a dynamic where they were either having sex or arguing.

Ryan was able to increase awareness of the way they avoided conflict and continued to isolate until they felt regulated and safe. They worked with an introjection from childhood, where their mother parentified them and told them they needed to save her from her pain. In rejection of this introjection, Ryan turned in on themselves and became the unfeeling one, as they wanted their mom to be. They could see that they projected this onto their partner, blaming Erin for the ways they (Ryan) agreed to do things they didn't want to do.

Exercise: 7 Steps to Alignment

This exercise is designed to support you in coming into full contact with yourself. The steps can easily be adapted to your work with clients (and are outlined in the workbook at the end of this book):

Step 1: Identify and Name

- ♦ To begin, close your eyes and bring your awareness to your current experience of yourself.
- ♦ Take a few breaths, and scan your mind and your body.
- ♦ Allow your attention to land on the loudest part of your inner world. This may be a thought in your mind or a sensation in your body.
- ♦ Name this aspect of your inner world.

Step 2: Witness

- ♦ Now that this aspect of you has been named, wrap it with awareness.
- ♦ Without trying to change this aspect of yourself and without trying to figure it out, allow yourself to be the loving witness.
- ♦ Let this part of you know that you see it.
- ♦ Say to this aspect of yourself, "I see you. I see that you are thinking/feeling ...."

Step 3: Validate

- ♦ Now that this aspect of you has been witnessed, validate it.
- ♦ Take a few breaths of validation and self-compassion.

♦ Say to this aspect of yourself, "It makes sense to me that you ...."
    ○ If this is a thought, validate the thought pattern.
♦ If this is an emotion, validate the emotional experience.

Step 4: Give It a Voice

♦ Now that this aspect of you has been validated, give it space to be heard.
♦ If this sensation or thought had a voice, what would it say?
    ○ With your words, speak from this aspect of yourself.
    ○ Use the first person. For example, if you're tending to tension in your jaw, perhaps your jaw says, "I can't let go."
♦ If you are tending to a thought pattern, perhaps the mind says, "I need to anticipate in order to stay safe."

Step 5: Be Curious

♦ Now that this aspect of you has spoken, be curious about it.
♦ As you sit in curiosity, is there anything you want to ask it?
♦ Why is it here?
♦ What does it need from you?
♦ Allow the answer to come forth to you.

Step 6: Open to Yourself

♦ Now that this aspect has been contacted, open to yourself.
♦ Give yourself what you need.
♦ Breathe in the breath of love, and allow your emotions to move through you.
♦ Honor what you have discovered about yourself.

Step 7: Honor Yourself

♦ From this place of openness to yourself, make a commitment to honor yourself.
♦ From contact with your needs, what are you willing to commit to yourself?
♦ Don't agree to anything you aren't fully ready to embody.
♦ For example, perhaps this aspect of yourself needed love. Your commitment may be, "I am ready to be more gentle with myself."
♦ Or perhaps, this aspect needed to feel safe. Your commitment may be, "I commit to listening to myself and discovering what I need to feel safe."

References

Naranjo, C. (2004). *Gestalt therapy: The attitude and practice of an atheoretical experientialism.* Crown House Pub Ltd.

Perls, F. (1973). *The Gestalt approach and eye witness to therapy* (1st ed.). Science and Behavior Books, Inc.

Polster, E., & Polster, M. (1973). *Gestalt therapy integrated: Contours of theory and practice.* Brunner/Mazel.

Yontef, G. (1993). *Awareness, dialogue & process: Essays on Gestalt therapy.* Gestalt Journal Press.

Yontef, G. (1998). Dialogic Gestalt therapy. In L. S. Greenberg, J. C. Watson, & G. Lietaer (Eds.), *Handbook of experiential psychotherapy* (pp. 82–102). The Guilford Press.

Chapter 14

Transpersonal Parts Work

Honoring the energetic consciousness being held in certain aspects of a client's personality, physical body, and subtle energy, we work in a transpersonal manner, where their innate spirituality is valued as the catalyst for their transformation. Through energetic attunement, awareness continuum, tending to the inner mind–body connection, and creative experimentation, clients explore the mystical realm of their humanity. Emphasizing the wholeness of who a client is as a multidimensional human being, we naturally explore *transpersonal parts work*. During these explorations, clients may encounter unexpected energies that are essential to their transformation, including sabotage patterns and energetic feeders.

Because these concepts are not widely spoken about in the world of psychology and psychotherapy, this chapter may seem too obscure to be practical. Understanding how to work with these patterns clinically, however, can support the client in stabilizing through memory consolidation, where an unstable memory is transformed into a steadier one (Dudai, 2004). When an imprint of a dark and distorted experience lives within the memory, working with it clinically offers clients a place to cultivate inner stability, clarity, and a sense of well-being. Processing the imprint through the mind, body, and subtle energy allows the client to clear what is toxic in their system in deep and lasting ways.

Aside from working with the malignant energy of toxic imprints, clients may encounter transpersonal allies as a resource in their process. Transpersonal allies include deceased loved ones, ancestors, and spirit guides. In the therapy room, to bring spirituality, consciousness, and subtle energy into the work is a revolutionary act of allowing process to supersede pathology. Working on the level of the mind is extremely important for increasing understanding, clarity, and choice. Working on the level of the body is extremely important for regulation, emotional processing, and integration. Working on the level of energy is profoundly effective in transmuting the deepest barriers to living in full alignment and returning to wholeness. The more practiced we become at attuning to subtle energy, the more we gain access to a new dimension of the therapeutic container.

This is a decolonized approach that is viewed as a normal part of healing in indigenous cultures (Talag, 2020). As with all experiments, transpersonal parts work is a practice of trial and error, where contact with the client is prioritized. Deferring to the client's awareness, insight, and deepest desire, we collaborate and engage with clients through the field of awareness (Clarkson & Caviccia, 2013). When the foundation of our clinical work is seated in the principles outlined up to this point, transpersonal parts work unfolds naturally, in

DOI: 10.4324/9781003521969-17

an intuitive and collaborative manner (Naranjo, 1978). The more we open to the awareness field and increase our intuitive sensitivities, the more apparent these transpersonal energies become. When they are recognized and acknowledged by the client, we can co-create experiments that offer a dynamic space for a client to move through the transpersonal dimensions of their inner psyche.

Energetic Attachment Cords

Energetic attachment cords are threads of spiritual and emotional connection with others that are formed in strong interpersonal connections (Brennan, 1988). In both healthy and unhealthy ways, attachment cords have us feel connected to others through the attachment system.

When these cords are healthy, they represent the secure attachment we have with another person. These cords, known as *aligned attachment cords*, are mutually beneficial connections that let both people know they are interconnected and entrusted with one another's well-being. With aligned attachment cords, each person is connected with their own boundless Source of energy. From this connection, attunement, love, and trust are co-created with the other person. These cords can be felt as an attachment bond, where we know that we are connected even when we're apart. In this exchange, neither person leaves contact with themselves to earn love and acceptance, nor do they disrupt contact with patterns of manipulation or blame. Both people feel more free and liberated for being attached in this way.

When attachment cords are an expression of a client's attachment wounds, they manifest as a *sabotage pattern* that reflects their unprocessed experiences from the past. Sabotage patterns are mental, physical, or subtle habits that interfere with a client's well-being and the health of their relationships. When a client has a low level of awareness and a high degree of developmental trauma, energetic movements of their attachment wounds can appear as sabotage patterns, affecting their behavior in relationships.

Unlike attachment cords, sabotage patterns are not mutually beneficial to relationships. Wounds guide the way a person engages in relationships when their sabotage patterns are being used. People use these patterns when they have forgotten that they have their own Source of energy and love within themselves, and they hyper-identify with patterns of attachment wounding, dependency, judgment, comparison, expectations, immaturity, and/or self-importance (Figure 14.1).

Here is a description of various sabotage patterns expressed through attachment cords:

♦ **Energetic Hooks** are used to reel another person in (either unconsciously or consciously). The energetic hook is intended to get another person's attention, to cause the other person to feel badly, and to have power over the other person. An energetic hook can be thrown by saying hurtful things, walking away in the midst of conflict, or giving a judgmental or demeaning glare.

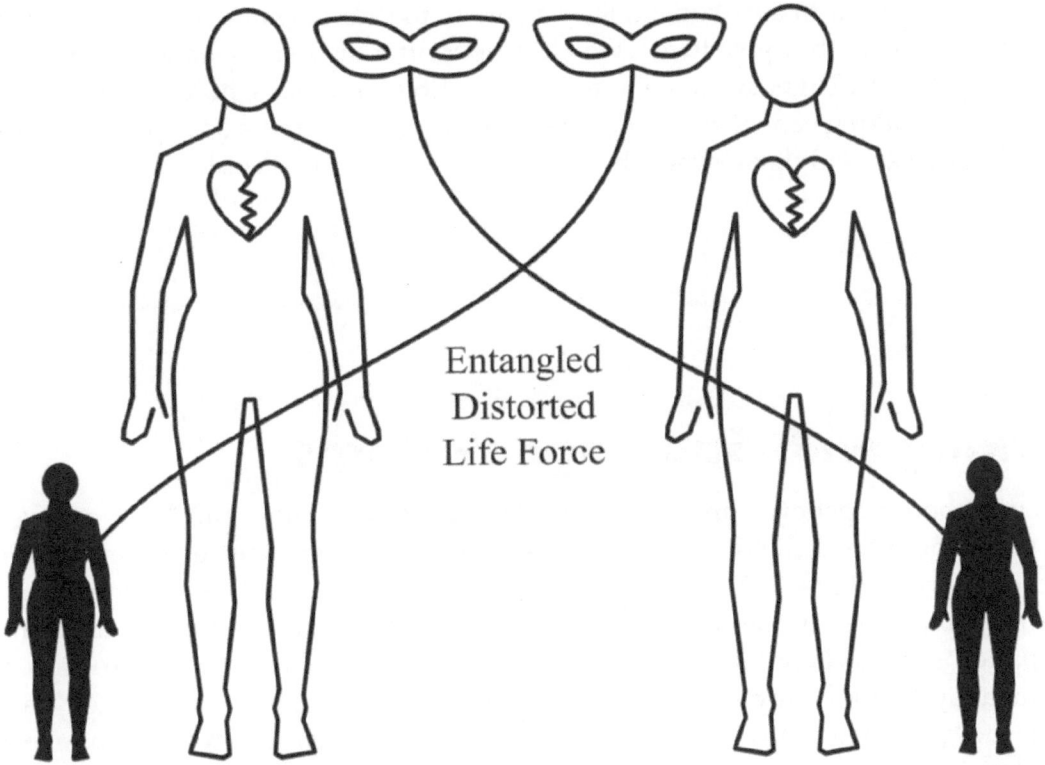

Figure 14.1 Relationship Entanglement (Kwiker, 2022, p. 180)

- **Energetic Feelers** are used to read another person in an attempt to control or manipulate them. Feelers are not the same as attunement, as they are used to read another in an effort to use the information they sense to influence the other. A person who uses feelers in an attempt to control typically was not offered healthy, safe attention and clear boundaries in early childhood development. They often needed to read other people in an effort to find safety.

- **Energetic Arrows** are used (either unconsciously or consciously) with the intention to hurt another person. Strategies of harming another person are used in an attempt to find a sense of power. The dark arrow can be thrown verbally, or it can be thrown energetically. When a person is hurting, and they don't have the awareness or ability to speak on behalf of their experience, they speak from their pain, and their words are hurtful, like an arrow. In psychology, we call this projective identification, which means that anything we are unwilling to feel in ourselves we unconsciously induce in others.

- **Energetic Suckers** are used when a person sucks the light from other people. This could be presented as loquacity, when the person takes up all the energy in the room. Some people refer to this as being an *energetic vampire*. In their presence, one can feel literally drawn in and lose access to oneself completely. When a person is dependent on other people for their sense of worth and okayness, they try to get energy from other people to give meaning to their life. The people in their life feel depleted and depressed being around them.

- **Energetic Siphon** is used when a person gives energy away, draining their own light to try to get approval, connection, and other forms of energy from others.

This can occur in a person who has a barrier to receiving and general codependent habits, where they give to get, which is siphoning their energy and creating an *energetic leak*. This makes them more susceptible to suckers, hooks, arrows, and probes. Taking care of everyone else's needs, treating others as more important than themselves, and disowning what they need are ways this could look in real time.

Working with Sabotage Patterns

Energetic sabotage patterns are seated in attachment wounding and have an overlay of projection, where the individual is denying something within themselves and assigning it to another person (Perls, 1973). Oftentimes, a client will see the dark attachment cords of a person in their life and be unable to see the way their system colludes with or matches those patterns. As a client talks about another person, we listen for the expression of their attachment system and any potential projections. Following the thread of their narratives back to the client, we can discover the client's sabotage patterns through the reflection of their relationships.

It is common for a client to have a specific sabotage pattern that colludes with the pattern of their partner. For example, a client may have a siphon sabotage pattern and is in relationship with a person who sucks their energy or throws dark arrows. Inviting the client to get energetic space from the other person allows them to explore repairing their energy leak, which is needed to be able to meet at the contact boundary.

Here are some ways to work with sabotage patterns:

♦ **Shadow work:** All people have both light and dark energy within us. What makes energy dark is that it lives in the shadow, which is the deep unconscious mind. To work with the shadow, illuminate your client's sabotage pattern by bringing it to the awareness field. Use neutral language that is not definitive. Then, think of an experiment that may help the client to increase awareness of their own shadow. Two-chair integration is useful in shadow work, where a client embodies their shadow by speaking from their sabotage pattern. Tremendous insight is gained in this process.

♦ **Reparenting:** Working with the inner young one is useful in getting to the place where the attachment injury occurred. Follow the thread of the pattern back to the first moment the client remembers feeling the way they feel in relationships. Work with healing the attachment wound and updating the young one.

♦ **Attaching to Self:** Support the client in connecting with their own needs and desires, and giving themselves what they think they want from others. Where the client wants others to be something for them, follow that thread back to the client, and support them in being that for themselves. Reparenting, empty chair, and two-chair are useful to increase awareness and find a way to attach to Self.

- ♦ **Clearing subtle energy:** Get the energy of the other person completely out of the room. If there is stickiness between them, you may need to support some type of containment, where the other person is in an imaginary crystal pyramid—then put them out of the room. Once the client is clear of the other person's energy, ask the client what they want for themselves in this moment. If their answer is about someone else, redirect them to themselves. How do they want to be? How do they want to show up? Their answer informs a potential experiment.

- ♦ **Cutting attachment cords:** Once you support the clearing of the client's energy, and they are attached to Self, any residual unhealthy threads between them and another person may become obvious. Ask the client what they want to do with the threads. If they want to cut them, invite them to do so lovingly.

- ♦ **Forgiveness:** Holding onto a resentment is an indicator of an unhealthy attachment cord. If the client is truly ready to let go of this attachment, ask them if they're interested in exploring a forgiveness practice. If they are, direct them to put the other person in an empty chair. Once they are there, ask them what words of forgiveness they genuinely want to say. If it seems helpful, you may want to offer the following: Invite them to repeat after you, "(Person's name), you've come into my life so that I may learn from you. I bless you and release you to your highest good elsewhere." Then, have them imagine the person surrounded in a golden light. "Go, be happy. I forgive you. Please forgive me, too."

- ♦ **Toning energetic boundaries:** Once the energy is clear and cords are cut, toning energetic boundaries is extremely important. When a client has a felt sense of their alignment, they can feel the fullness of their energy body. This fullness is what creates a toned boundary system. Invite the client to put one hand in front of them like a stop sign and then tap their sternum with the fingertips of their other hand. Then, have them imagine the other person is sitting in front of them, and have them say, "I am here, and you are there." Have them repeat this several times, then remind them that any time this person thinks of them, it bounces off of their energetic boundary, and they get redirected to the Source that beats their heart. Any time they think of this person, they get redirected to Source.

Energetic Feeders

Through the lens of the transpersonal, the qualities that we see in others are not separate from ourselves. This is a non-dual philosophy that sees unification as the ultimate reality (Spira, 2022). Separation is viewed as an illusion, and we honor our interconnectedness with all of life. This is the essence of True Self awareness, and when it arises from an authentic place, it is a sacred expression of innate spirituality. When there are elements in the environment that are toxic, however, a client must differentiate from these elements in order to process an experience and make contact with themselves. A toxic energy, such as an entity that feeds off of the person's vital force, is considered an introjection. An introjection is defined as "alien accretions [that] are added to the personality" (Perls, 1973).

When a toxic force enters into the client's mind, body, and energy, it causes an overall instability that is persistent and troublesome. Entities enter into a person's psyche, body, and energy during moments of trauma and dissociation. For example, a child could have acquired an entity from a caregiver who was a violent alcoholic and sexually abusive. Because the experience was too big, too confusing, and too violating to fully digest, their psyche holds a memory imprint of a dark, toxic force. To survive this experience, they adapt by organizing their personality around the introjected entity. Their physical body and their subtle energy store this introject as well.

> People grow through biting off an appropriate-sized piece (be this food or ideas or relationships), chewing it (considering), and discovering whether it is nourishing or toxic. If nourishing, the organism assimilates it and makes it part of itself. If toxic, the organism spits it out (rejects it). This requires people to be willing to trust their taste and judgment. Discrimination requires *actively* sensing outside stimuli and processing these exteroceptive stimuli along with interoceptive data.
>
> (Yontef, 1993)

Working to support the client in differentiating from the dark, toxic introjection allows memory consolidation, a process by which they rediscover their inner stability. As the toxic introjection is moved out, their soul fully finds its seat in their body, supporting full embodiment. And when this dark force is cleared from their energy body, the client is able to find their way back to spiritual alignment, where the parasitic introject no longer depletes their vital force and they are guided by their innate spirituality.

Toxic energies tend to hang out in the places with the most emotional energy pollution (EEP). They can latch on during dissociative trauma, and they can come into a person's field during dissociative drug and alcohol experiences. Since they feed off people's vital force, they glom onto people with the most open systems.

There are a few characteristics that a client might display that indicate this work could be useful: They are continually antagonistic with themselves; they dissociate; they demonstrate sabotage patterns, where they inhibit their own personal progress; they are cruel to those closest to them; their caregivers were cruel to them, and they cannot bear the pain of their past; their energy is chronically collapsed, dark, and weak. There may be other presentations; however, it is important to note that this is not the same symptom presentation as psychosis. In order to do this work, a client must have enough inner resources to be with it consciously; otherwise, there is a risk of destabilizing a client who actually needs more inner resourcing and less inner disruption.

Working with an energetic feeder is similar to the way we work with other introjections, via an empty chair experiment. By getting space from the introjection and putting it into a chair, the client's innate wisdom and intuition will be the true guide in what unfolds. It is neither important nor relevant that we know if we are working with an entity, nor do we name it as such. Similarly, the client doesn't need to know if it's an entity to move this energy. Facilitating an empty chair experiment with the introjection is enough to be with the toxic energy consciously.

As the experiment begins, and the client attempts to put the introjection in a chair, they may describe it in the following ways: It's *sticky*, like tar. It's *slippery*, like oil. It's *long and hairy*, like a clogged pipe. This is an indicator that we are working with toxic energy that has been acquired and has been keeping them imbalanced.

♦ To begin the experiment, instruct the client to put the introjection into a chair. Have them use their hands to remove the introjection and place it in the chair. As they do this, they may say, "It's so slippery. I can't get it. It keeps slipping through my fingers." Or they may say, "It's so sticky. I can't get it off of me." Or, "It's so long and hairy. It's like a snake coming out of my throat, but it doesn't end."

♦ In these moments, the client's sovereign will is needed to get the entity completely out of their energy body. Support them in finding the inner strength to remove the introjection. If they seem collapsed around their will, you may ask them if they want help, and you can use your words, awareness, and movement to remove the energy from their field. Alternatively, you can ask them if they'd like to call on any helpers or guides that they are connected to.

♦ In order to differentiate from the entity, take your time and invite the client's awareness to fully occupy their inner world. The more they occupy their entire being and body, the less room there is for energy that doesn't belong to them. The more sovereign will they have access to, the more choice they have about what is allowed within them.

♦ Once they get the entity out of their energy body, slow down and invite them to deepen into their body. Ask the client what they notice and if there is anything they want to say to the introjection. A question like "Why are you here?" or a statement like "It's time for you to go" can often be enough to have the entity move on.

♦ You might also ask the client if there is anything they want to do with the entity. Common ideas are putting it in a fire or a crystal pyramid. This happens in the energetic field.

♦ It is not important or recommended for the client to sit in the seat of the toxic energy. If they want to, this is their choice. However, clients typically want the energy gone and would rather not sit in it now that it is finally out of their system.

Deceased Loved Ones

When a client is grieving or has unfinished business with a deceased loved one, it can be helpful to experiment with inviting that loved one into the room. As the consciousness of the loved one lives on in the spirit realm, they can be allies in the client's healing. When we are open to the intuitive field, we are able to sense and hear the consciousness of the deceased loved one. This is also true for the client when they are open to the awareness field that can feel and hear the consciousness of those who have crossed over.

♦ An accessible way to work with a deceased loved one is by asking the client, "If they were here right now, what would you say to them?" An intuitive dialogue can unfold naturally from here. Follow the client's lead on what they hear and experience in the conversation. If you hear the voice of the deceased loved one, share the insight gained in a neutral way: "I think I'm hearing it as …." Honor your intuitive ability without crossing the sacred boundary and putting it onto the client.

♦ Another way to work with a deceased loved one is through an empty chair experiment. Inviting the loved one into the room offers the client an opportunity to speak to their loved one. They may be able to hear their response and message from their own seat, or they may want to move to the chair of the loved one to hear and feel their consciousness. If they move chairs, they will likely feel and hear the presence of the loved one, making the transmission more accessible for them.

Ancestral Lineage

Ancestral healing can release the weight of family patterns and support the repair of the epigenetics, where a client's familial genes that have been altered through stress, trauma, and other distressing circumstances can be restored. Working with ancestral patterns is a sacred process by which we honor the wisdom of the client and the ancestors while gently facilitating a repair in the lineage. Clients have the opportunity to be the catalyst for change, where certain sabotage patterns or limiting values that hold them back can be transmuted for themselves and future generations.

In many cases, a client may seek to understand how the pain and trauma of their ancestors affected them and come in with a desire to work on their lineage patterns. Alternatively, either you or the client may have a spontaneous insight or epiphany about how their mental and emotional constructs have been passed through generations. When it is known that a client wants to work with their ancestral lineage, we can offer the work through a visualization or an empty chair:

♦ **Visualization:** Invite the client to sense all the way back to where this pattern emerged in their lineage. They may have a memory of their parent or grandparent, which is a good place to start. Have them see that ancestor and then continue to look back even farther to the ancestors they never met. Invite them to see those ancestors who adapted to their environment by creating this pattern. See if the client can sense the lack of resources, systems oppression, or misuse of power that precipitated the pattern.
  ○ Ask the client if there is anything they are hearing or sensing from the ancestor.
  ○ Ask the client if there is anything they want to ask or say to their ancestor.
  ○ Ask the client what is needed to transmute this pattern. The wisdom and guidance ancestors can offer can support the repair of the lineage pattern.
  ○ When and if appropriate, invite the client to feel the support of their ancestors. This support is typically offered to their back, as ancestors are behind the client.

- When and if appropriate, invite the client to sense into the future generations in front of them. Invite them to feel their entire lineage pattern, including where they are in the line.
- **Empty Chair:** Invite the client to place their ancestors in the empty chair. This can be one ancestor or all ancestors. It is up to the client to decide.
  - Ask the client how their ancestor(s) seem to them. What do they look like energetically?
  - Ask the client if there is anything they want to ask or say to their ancestor(s).
  - Ask the client if there is anything they are hearing or sensing from the ancestor(s).
  - Ask the client what is needed to transmute this pattern. Invite the wisdom and guidance of the ancestors to offer support for the repair of the lineage pattern.
  - Ask the client if there is anything they want to say or ask about the pattern in the lineage they are shifting.
  - Ask the client if there is anything else needed in relationship to their ancestor(s) in order to complete this pattern.

Spirit Guides

When a therapist and a client open into awareness, we're collaboratively listening to alternate dimensions, which offers the client insight and understanding that serves their healing. When the therapist and the client intentionally ask for support from those alternate dimensions, a client can gain resources that serve their healing.

Every once in a while, when a client feels stuck and incapable of moving a deep energetic pattern, it can be useful to offer that the client invites their spirit guides to support them. Not all clients feel connected with their spirit guides, and they may not be interested in receiving support from these alternate dimensions. Because of this, it is important to know your client's world-view and cultural lens before offering the invitation of asking for transpersonal support.

When a client is interested, it is important to ask them what guides in the spirit realm they relate to. Some clients resonate with the language of helpers or angels, while others resonate with fairies or guides. Some resonate with Buddha Nature or Divine Spirit, while others resonate with a deceased loved one or ancestors.

Having allies in the spirit realm is often overlooked as an accessible resource. When and if we decide to offer our clients the invitation, we must do so with a sense of neutrality and non-attachment. The most important aspect of working with spirit guides is that clients decide if this happens, and they decide what guides they feel connected with. The surrender a client experiences when they allow their helpers to support them in their healing is healing in and of itself.

Transcript: Cutting Cords

The client arrived to the session talking about a relationship that they wanted to set some boundaries in. It was not an intimate relationship, but it was a relationship that they could not fully sever or end for many reasons. They could feel energetic cords with this person and wanted them to be cut. I began by inviting the client to turn toward the cords and witness them in an effort to contact them and learn from them before we tried an experiment.

CLIENT: The cords feel toxic and they don't belong here. I don't feel safe when they're here. It's not healthy for me.

THERAPIST: What do you notice when you say that?

CLIENT: The truth of those words resonate deeply. And I am also in touch with anger and disappointment that I allowed it.

THERAPIST: Anger and disappointment that you allowed it. What do you notice when you say that?

CLIENT: Softening and some compassion. But I want to get rid of them.

THERAPIST: Ok. If it's okay with you, let's get this person who you have these cords with completely out of the room. Sending them back to wherever they are. (Silence)

CLIENT: It's hard to do because it's not far enough and the cording is still there.

THERAPIST: Yeah. I feel that. Just notice that. That even with distance you're still connected with the cords. What do you notice?

CLIENT: Tightness.

THERAPIST: If that tightness had a voice, what would it say?

CLIENT: Help me. (Tears) I feel sad.

THERAPIST: Make room for the sadness. (Notice that I am not rescuing the client, but instead supporting them in increasing awareness on their way to their autonomy.) How far away do you want them?

CLIENT: A different planet. (This is a common response.)

THERAPIST: What do you notice when you say that?

CLIENT: I feel lighter.

THERAPIST: Notice that lightness and notice how much room that makes for you. What do you notice?

CLIENT: The cord feels thinner because it's so stretched out, so it feels easier to imagine not being so plugged in. (This is a common experience and useful in finding their way back to themselves.)

THERAPIST: What do you notice in your belly? (This is where the cords live, so I want to check in here.)

CLIENT: Discomfort, but not too bad.

THERAPIST: I want to invite you to keep shining the light of awareness on your belly. Keep occupying that space fully. (The intention here is to fill the cord area with the client's consciousness, which is essential in getting other people's energy out.) What do you notice now?

CLIENT: That prompt offers me a sense of "Mine" and I keep breathing into that.

THERAPIST: Yes! This is your space. Beautiful. (Silence) What do you notice now?

CLIENT: Calm and aware and patient.

THERAPIST: I find myself wanting to hear the words from you about what you want for yourself right now. (Even though it may seem obvious, it's important that the client's desire is named with clarity to guide what we do next.)

CLIENT: I want less of a trigger in me around this person when they blatantly attack me and throw dark cords. And I want to stop feeling on edge anticipating their attack. I want a sense of neutrality and freedom from this.

THERAPIST: Slowing down and feeling the truth of what you want. Neutrality and freedom.

CLIENT: And there's fear that it's not possible.

THERAPIST: Noticing that fear is here. Welcoming the full range of your experience.

The client felt tension and sadness, and cried many tears. They also touched into wanting the other person to be different, and wanted to feel free even if the other person didn't change. They could also see how they trapped themselves by being guarded, but they did not want to let their guard down.

THERAPIST: Noticing your connection to your home base, the core of your being up the midline of your body.

CLIENT: Interesting, I just had this sense of resource from my partner show up, and realizing that I can create that internally here within myself.

THERAPIST: What do you notice in your body?

CLIENT: Strength and uprightness.

THERAPIST: And feel that in your body, that this strength is yours.

CLIENT: As you say that I can feel this hole in my gut, this place that is lacking that truth. (This is where they give their power away and allow the cords in.)

THERAPIST: Noticing where the strength is, first. We'll come back to the empty space in a moment, but notice where you do feel strong. What do you notice when you tend to that?

CLIENT: Feeling tearful at the power of myself and my heart.

THERAPIST: A few more breaths here, feeling your power. And from your heart, notice how that is also connected down to your belly and to your navel. What do you notice there?

CLIENT: It's hard to connect … (breathes) … (cries) … like a wire got cut from my heart to my root.

THERAPIST: And as you let the tears come, keep seeing the wire. I'm wondering if there is anything it needs from you right now?

CLIENT: (Cries, breathes, and subtle energy moves in tremendous ways) It wants connection and repair. Connection within myself. I can see these tendrils of light that are reaching towards one another, coming back.

THERAPIST: Staying there, connecting and repairing with the tendrils of light.

CLIENT: It's like in Avatar, where the beings connect with the trees.

THERAPIST: Beautiful. Keep seeing that inherent wisdom in your body. That movement towards health and healing. (Silence) What do you notice now?

CLIENT: There's a connection. It's internal in the center of my body. It feels really good and strong. It's not a hole anymore.

THERAPIST: Stay there as you really see that connection and occupying that space within you that is yours. All the way down through your root, connecting all the way down. What do you notice there?

CLIENT: It's getting thicker, and it's very lit up.

THERAPIST: A few breaths up and down the midline, really tending to and connecting with your home base. Landing there in your root, your seat of safety and security right there in your own body. From this place, I'm noticing the desire to support you in unhooking the cords. What do you notice when I say that?

CLIENT: Yes, absolutely.

THERAPIST: I want to invite you to use your words and your hands to unhook. What would you say to this person about this hook as you take it from you …?

CLIENT: With my hands, it does feel like a hook, so I'm going to move that and throw it to the planet they are on. This isn't mine. You don't belong here. You can't touch me … which is shaky and hard to say.

THERAPIST: Noticing it's shaky, but I'm wondering is it true?

CLIENT: Yes, it's true.

THERAPIST: What do you notice?

CLIENT: Anger.

THERAPIST: Let me hear from anger as you unhook.

CLIENT: I want to scream.

THERAPIST: Scream. (Therapist groans) No!

CLIENT: (Screams) No … You don't belong here. Yeah … I feel that. This is my space.

THERAPIST: Stay with that. And if you have access to any helpers or guides you connect with, you can invite them to support you, too.

CLIENT: I feel so clear and so much more space. I feel like I'm detoxing.

Lessons from the Therapy Room

Early in my career, I studied a technique called Trauma Resilience Model (TRM). Learning a model of working with trauma that aligned with gestalt principles eased my apprehension and fear around my own inadequacies. I learned how to frontload clients with inner resources and co-regulate with them during their traumatic stress reactions. I also learned how to create experiments that support the client's deepest healing and shift in the way they relate to the trauma.

Around this time, I started to work with a client who had been sexually assaulted multiple times. One of the assaults she had endured occurred when she was drugged and gang raped. All these incidents had happened many years ago, and she had already experienced many years of therapy. She came to me looking for a deeper and more holistic approach to working with her trauma.

Uncertain about what would unfold, I followed the TRM protocol and began by frontloading her with a resource. She recalled a memory of a time when she felt safe in a meadow near her hometown. We amplified that resource by having her sense into the temperature, sounds, and smells associated with that memory. As her body began to receive that memory, her muscles relaxed, and she appeared tranquil.

After a few moments, I invited her to tell me about the assault. Because she had been drugged, the memory of the violence was not an active one. She remembered waking up and feeling a burning pain in her genitals, and then instantly seeing the face of a man who had been pestering her the night before. She then went on to recall the days that followed when she put together what had happened, as melancholy began to set in.

Because her system was entrained to be in hypo-arousal, her level of activation seemed low as she recalled this memory. I invited her to come back to the meadow where she felt safe, and I guided her in accessing the felt sense of that safety. Her freeze response began to melt, as she looked like she was coming back to life. Titrating between her resource and the memory, she was able to stay within her window of tolerance, where there was enough activation to work with and enough resource to make this a healing experience.

I invited her to come back to the memory of the trauma, and she sensed the predator in the room, who she described as the ring leader to the other perpetrators. She froze and became immobile, and it was as if the drug were in her system again. When I asked her what she wanted to do with the predator, she responded, "I want him out but he won't leave." She described the darkness in her genitals, which was his energy living in her system.

"I need you to help," she said.

At that request, I stood up and said, "Leave. Get out. You can't hurt her anymore. Get out!" I opened the door and moved his energy out. The freeze in her system began to thaw, and the color started to come back to her face. She started to use her hands to clear him out of her energy body, and I kept helping by moving him all the way out.

She thanked me and said she'd been needing that help for a long time. "I don't want him out there hurting other people," she said.

"What would you like to do with him?" I asked.

She silently contemplated that for several minutes. "I want to put him in a box and seal him in." I invited her to see that in her mind's eye. "But now I don't know what to do with the box. Maybe I can put him in the ocean, far away from any people."

We sat in silence as she did that. Slowly, she seemed more relaxed and alert. This was my first encounter with transpersonal parts work, but it wasn't my last. The discovery process of co-creating a session with the client is so dynamic and creative. Never knowing what part of a client's inner world is going to reveal itself, each session offers new opportunities for clients to complete unfinished business and deepen into themselves.

Exercise: Forgiveness Practice

When a client is fully present and awake, it is common for them to naturally find their way to forgiveness. Other times, the client may have a more challenging time fully letting go of sabotage patterns and forgiving themselves and others for harm caused. This forgiveness practice at the end of the session, invited with consent of the client, can truly support a shift in perspective.

As with any experiment, we begin by asking the client if they are open to trying something. If they are, we let them know that we are thinking about trying a forgiveness practice. If they are still interested, we proceed.

Have the client close their eyes and imagine the person they resent or who harmed them. Then, slowly, ask them to say the following to the person:

"(Person's name), you've come into my life so that I may learn from you. I bless you and release you to your highest good elsewhere."

Then have them envision the person surrounded in divine light, and say, "Go. Be happy. I forgive you. Please forgive me, too."

Then invite them to let that person go to their highest good elsewhere. Use the awareness continuum to check in with how that was for them, and then, ask them if they want to do that for themselves, too. This is especially powerful if they are mad at themselves for past decisions and actions.

If they want to try this, have them imagine the younger version of themselves. This is the part of them that made those decisions. And have them repeat after you:

"(Client's name), you've come into my life so that I may learn from you. I bless you and release you to your highest good elsewhere."

Then have them envision the younger version of themselves surrounded in divine light, and say, "Go. Be happy. I forgive you. Please forgive me, too."

References

Brennan, B. (1988). *Hands of light: A guide to healing through the human energy field* (Reissue ed.). Bantam.

Clarkson, P., & Caviccia, S. (2013). *Gestalt counselling in action.* Sage Publications.

Dudai, Y. (2004). The neurobiology of consolidations, or, how stable is the engram? *Annual Review of Psychology, 55,* 51–86.

Kwiker, H. (2022). *Align: Living and loving from the true self.* Mantra Books.

Naranjo, C. (1978). Gestalt therapy as a transpersonal approach. *Gestalt Journal, 1*(2), 75–81.

Perls, F. (1973). *The Gestalt approach and eye witness to therapy* (1st ed.). Science and Behavior Books, Inc.

Spira, R. (2022). *You are the happiness you seek: Uncovering the awareness of being.* Sahaja Press.

Talag, T. (2020). *All Our relations: Indigenous trauma in the shadow of colonialism.* Scribe Publications.

Yontef, G. (1993). Chapter 6 - Gestalt Therapy - Clinical Phenomenology. *Awareness, Dialogue and Process - Essays on Gestalt Therapy.* NY: The Gestalt Journal Press, 181–201.

Chapter 15

Working with Dreams and Other Non-Ordinary States

Non-ordinary states of consciousness are unique perceptions, thoughts, and emotions that are typically not accessible from an ordinary level of awareness (Aixala & Bouso, 2022). Experiences of non-ordinary awareness are temporary, and they can be aided by an external source or created organically through contemplative practices. Common ways consciousness is altered include dreaming, meditation, hypnosis, breathwork, psychedelics, or plant medicine. Sometimes, an altered reality can be distressing, such as sleep deprivation, psychosis, or a negative side effect of psychoactive drugs. However, when a person is intentional with their non-ordinary states and enters into them in a safe way, these experiences can be extremely healing, offering spiritual insights and enhanced creativity.

Entering into non-ordinary states of consciousness can be profound and transformative. Through meditation, for example, a person can practice differentiating from their ordinary mind and arrive into a dimension of their being that they normally overlook. Mystical experiences such as expansion into universal wisdom, infinite love, healing, and unification with all of life emerge naturally from the awakened brain.

Revering non-ordinary states as sacred helps to safeguard a practitioner from inserting their ego into the offerings of these transcendent gifts. Continuing the example of meditation, a person's ego may want to bottle up the mystical experience and keep it forever. This impulse adulterates the experience and taints its purity. Stepping out of the way and being present to the innate wisdom and sacred healing powers of non-ordinary states supports the container to be held with devotion.

Dream Work

The most common non-ordinary state is dreaming. It is a rare individual who does not experience a dream state while sleeping, which occurs during the sleep cycle called *rapid eye movement* (REM). REM sleep deprivation disrupts the brain's ability to generate new cells, illustrating how important this non-ordinary state of consciousness is for the health of the brain (Blumberg et al. 2020).

DOI: 10.4324/9781003521969-18

Research has found (Peever & Fuller, 2017) that

key emotional and memory-related structures of the brain are reactivated during REM sleep as we dream. This means that emotional memory reactivation is occurring in a brain free of a key stress chemical, which allows us to re-process upsetting memories in a safer, calmer environment.

Working with dreams in a therapeutic session provides the client with a sacred container to discover what emotional and memory content they were processing during a dream. This makes it possible to integrate that content in a deeply embodied way, where it can be a healing influence on their ordinary, waking state.

Across various therapy theories (Beck, 2002; Freud, 2010; Perls, 1992; Jung, 1909), dreams are explored as a representation of the client's deepest subconscious mind. Many therapeutic approaches position the therapist as the expert who interprets or analyzes the dream. The therapist may even use dream symbols and try to decode their meanings for the client.

The gestalt approach to working with dreams is much dynamic and interesting. Instead of dissecting the dream, we bring it to life in the here and now (Perls, 1992). The dream is viewed as a landscape for the client to enact certain aspects of their inner subconscious. The places within a client's personality that they have disowned, avoided, or been afraid to look at are what they embody and become through the course of a dream work session.

In the dream itself, it becomes evident that the client's subconscious projects their own thoughts and emotions onto another person, object, substance, or place. By becoming each element of the dream, the client embodies the consciousness of that component. As we create a space for the client to feel and experience each part of the dream, they gain insight into an essential message from their psyche about their existence.

In this way, clients discover the meaning of their dreams for themselves as they are guided by presence and awareness. As we honor the dream as a sacred representation of the client's inner life, we follow and trust the client's deep inner knowing. While holding to all the therapeutic tenets already described in this book, we also point out the places in the dream that the client may be avoiding or overlooking.

Dream work is a profound experiment, offering clients a space to dive deeper into their existential experience. Some clients mention dreams as a quick aside. Other clients are really curious about their dreams and see them as significant. Either way, if we decide to offer the opportunity to work with a dream, we present it as an experiment: "Would you like to try something with this dream?"

- If the client is interested, ask them to describe the dream from their perspective in the present moment as if it's happening. For example: "I am standing in a graveyard. It's night, but I can see the words inscribed on the tombstones …. I think one belongs to my ancestor … I see the night guard coming …."
  - Weave in reflective listening and the awareness continuum, making room for the client to recall and express the dream in its entirety. Ask them present moment questions to support their deepening into the dream-land.
  - As you listen, note significant symbols in the dream, such as people, objects, substances, structures, and so on.
- Next, invite the client to describe the dream from a different perspective. You may want to suggest a significant symbol for them to become, or they may choose it

themselves. The invitation is to speak from this alternate perspective in the present moment from the first person. "I am the tombstone. (Client's name) is looking at me … They seem confused and scared. I'm here always, a steady presence pointing to (client's name) ancestors …."

- As they're talking from this element, ask them questions to support the filling out of the dream and increasing of awareness. For example, you might ask, "How do you feel as you see (client's name)?"

♦ Once that is complete, direct the dream theater experiment as the client continues to become the various elements of the dream. They will continue to speak from the first person as if it were happening in the present moment, and they may need your support in staying with this specific language.

- You can ask them what aspect of the dream they'd like to become next, and/or you can suggest an element that seems important. For example, they may become the grave itself. Then, they may become the night guard. Then, the lamp post. Then, the graveyard.

♦ Invite the client to become all of the main elements of the dream to fill out the entire landscape as much as possible. If there was a house or building involved, it is recommended to save that for the final symbol, as it often provides clients with a space to contact their witness mind and greater awareness.

- The client discovers deep insight in this process, and it inevitably changes the way they relate to and understand the dream.

♦ Once all of the elements of the dream have been embodied, invite the client to return to their original perspective and talk through the dream again from themselves.

- Direct them to talk through the entire dream again, in the first person, as if it were currently happening. However, this time, invite them to describe the dream as they would like it to unfold.

- This is a profound and empowering experience that gives the client insight into who they are and how they relate to the environment.

- If the dream is a nightmare and/or there's a point of powerlessness in the dream, take note of how they describe this in the final round of completing in the dream. They may need your support and guidance in finding their inner power to fully complete the dream.

Breathwork

Breathwork is an ancient breathing technique that originates from the lineage of Kriya Yoga, as passed down to the West from Haidakhan Babaji of India (Orr, 2013). In a breathwork session, a person practices conscious connected breathing, where they breathe in and out of the nose *or* in and out of the mouth, without stopping at the top or the bottom of the breath. This technique activates the self-cleaning mechanism of the breath, allowing higher levels of consciousness to intuitively move through the breath and into tension patterns (Fincham et al., 2023). Any emotional energy pollution (EEP) being held in the physical, emotional, and energetic bodies is transmuted with the vital healing energy of the breath.

Conscious connecting breathwork takes a person on a journey from ordinary awareness of separation, limitation, and suffering into non-ordinary states of expansion, transcendence, and healing. Opening to the breath in this way has been found to be effective in decreasing anxiety, increasing tranquility, and supporting a person's physical, mental, and spiritual well-being (Montes & Penzenstadler, 2023). Mystical experiences frequently transpire, where the mind becomes clear, old trauma is resolved, and spirituality unifies the wholeness of one's being.

Breathwork offers us a means of self-knowledge, where awareness, vital force, and devotion to Divinity reset the nervous system in a deeply embodied way. Emotional energy pollution and psychic dirt are cleared from the system, and a person feels a sense of interconnectedness with all of life. Increased intuition, creativity, and openheartedness can emerge from a single breathwork session.

Overall, breathwork is a powerful way to explore non-ordinary states of consciousness, where we can experience a deeper sense of connection to ourselves and the world. Therapeutically, however, this is not an intervention we offer to clients. If clients are interested, they can seek out a breathwork practitioner separate from the work we do with them. However, we can be a resource to support them in assimilating the experience, where the epiphanies and breakthroughs they have in a breathwork session are integrated through our work. This supports a client in bringing the lessons from the non-ordinary state into their life in a practical way.

Even though breathwork is not a clinical modality, we can certainly benefit from using it as a self-care tool. When a therapist clears their energy body with the power of conscious connected breathing, they are better equipped to hold space for clients. When we cultivate inner spaciousness through breathwork, the container we hold becomes a spacious place for clients to explore their inner world. When we are practiced with non-ordinary states, opening to the transformative power of awareness in a session becomes more accessible. From this benevolent place within, we embody what it means to be a healer, where our presence reminds others they are already whole.

Psychedelic Integration

Psychedelic assisted therapy is the therapeutic use of hallucinogenic substances administered in a safe container with a certified clinician. In most cases, synthetic substances, such as ketamine and methylenedioxymethamphetamine (MDMA), are prescribed and administered on site at a clinic. In other instances, naturally occurring plant medicine, such as psilocybin containing mushrooms, is used in either an individual or a group setting.

MDMA has been found effective to treat Post-Traumatic Stress Disorder (PTSD), and ketamine has been found effective for treatment-resistant depression (Parrot, 2014; Strong &

Kabbaj, 2018). With these synthetic hallucinogens, there are potential dangers to be aware of. In the case of MDMA, there is a period of time after administration where a client experiences "neurochemical recovery, when low serotonin levels are often accompanied by lethargy and depression" (Parrott, 2014). With ketamine, there are "potential addictive and cognitive-impairing effects of repeated ketamine infusions" (Strong & Kabbaj, 2018).

Plant medicines, such as psilocybin mushrooms, are gaining therapeutic interest for their unique ability to treat substance abuse disorders, post-traumatic stress, generalized anxiety, and clinical depression (Ziff et al., 2022). Research (Mortaheb et al., 2024) using brain imaging has shown that psilocybin "generates profound alterations both at the brain and experiential levels."

As a serotonin receptor agonist, psilocybin binds to and stimulates serotonin receptors, resetting the default mode network, which is a set of functionally interconnected brain regions that are responsible for a person's sense of identity (Mortaheb et al., 2024). Brain regions that normally wouldn't communicate with one another begin to communicate, creating an ability for the brain to rewire default modes and recreate a sense of identity. Neurotrophic factors, which are a "group of proteins that play a critical role in the growth, survival and maintenance of neurons," initiate a sense of *oceanic boundlessness* (Ziff et al., 2022). This hyperconnectivity of brain activity is present in spiritual experiences, including blissfulness, access to inherent wisdom, and unity with all of creation.

Indigenous cultures have been harnessing the healing powers of plant medicines for tens of thousands of years (Bruhn et al., 2002). They have been found to offer mystical-type experiences, with substantial and sustained personal meaning and spiritual significance, as well as a high degree of safety and enduring positive effects (Szigeti et al., 2024). The curative properties of plants cannot be fully reproduced in a lab, as they are a sacred offering from the earth.

Unlike synthetic substances, the naturally occurring hallucinogen psilocybin has been found to have low toxicity levels, a low risk of overuse, and minimal side effects (Ziff et al., 2022). A medical side effect of psychedelics is an elevation in blood pressure and heart rate (Frecska, 2007). While this is safe for most people, those who have a seizure disorder or severe cardiovascular disease should consult a physician before exploring psychedelic assisted therapies. Similarly, because psychedelics work by activating serotonin receptors, they are contraindicated for people using SSRI (selective serotonin reuptake inhibitors) and MAO-I (monoamine oxidase inhibitor) antidepressants. A rare side-effect of psychedelic use is prolonged psychosis, and therefore, it is contraindicated for individuals who have been diagnosed with schizophrenia, schizoaffective disorder, or bipolar 1 disorder (Frecska, 2007).

Non-ordinary states supported by synthetic hallucinogens or plant medicine offer new dimensions of healing for those who seek these medicines. While therapists are required to have state-specific certifications to offer psychedelic assisted therapy, any therapist with interest and knowledge can support a client in their integration. Psychedelic integration is defined as "implementing and incorporating the key insights and awareness gained in the psychedelic experience into their life" (Gorman et al., 2021). Integration is a process by which a client takes the time to understand what their psychedelic experience revealed to them. This process helps clients expand their awareness to create lasting changes.

In indigenous cultures, integration is built into the sacred rituals that are offered before, during, and after a plant medicine journey.

In order to address imbalance and support the realignment of self, shamanic cultures may employ symbolism and rituals already entrenched in the culture, such as hypnosis or trance-like states, drumming, chanting, spirit manifestations, among others, all within a communal context, which stimulate engagement with the innate drive toward physiological, spiritual and social experiences. (Aixala, 2017)

In Western cultures, integration is often influenced by "binaries that polarize and compartmentalize our thinking, for example, mind and body, self and other, or person and nature" (Barker & Lantaffi, 2019). There is a need to support clients in integrating their psychedelic experiences, not just after they journeyed but through every step along the way. The process of integration bridges the awareness gained through the psychedelic experience into their ordinary awareness, exploring new perspectives and possibilities. Integration work can support a client in working toward understanding and releasing emotional pain. It also helps them to gain clarity about how their mind constructs obstacles that contribute to their suffering. The insight and mystical awareness that gather during a psychedelic journey are just the beginning of their transformation. How they bring this new awareness with them into everyday life is where true transformation occurs.

To maximize the benefits of their experience, there are various practices a client can do to synthesize their inner mind–body experience throughout the entire journey of exploring a non-ordinary state of consciousness.

Here are some practices that support psychedelic integration *before* and *during* the journey:

♦ If the client has any risk factors, such as cardiovascular disease, disease of the liver, seizure disorder, severe suicidal ideation, psychosis, schizophrenia, or bipolar disorder, encourage them to seek medical advice before ingesting the medicine.

♦ If they have these above conditions, ask them if their facilitator is trained in working with these risk factors.

♦ If they take prescribed lithium, antipsychotics, or psychotropics, ask them if their facilitator is educated in these medications.

♦ Encourage them to eat nourishing foods that are low in salt, such as fresh fruit and veggies. Good food supports the digestion of the medicine.

♦ Before a journey, support the client in getting clear about their intention for entering into this non-ordinary state. What are they ready to transform and transmute? What are they ready to open to within themselves?

♦ Before a journey, support them in anchoring into their breath as a resource to come back to throughout the journey. What other resources do they want to have as an anchor? Is there a sacred item they want to bring with them or an altar they want to make?

♦ What items would make them more comfortable during the journey? Preparing by making a nest with a fuzzy blanket, pillow, and water bottle is an act of self-care that can nurture them throughout the experience.

Here are some practices that support psychedelic integration *after* the journey:

♦ Encourage them to have nourishing food available for after the journey, such as fresh fruit and veggies. Good food is really important for integration, in that it supports the ongoing intention of being healthy and vital.

- Encourage them to explore movement practices, such as dance and yoga. Moving in a way that feels joyful and delicious to the body supports deeper embodiment after the journey.
- Invite them to draw an artistic representation of the journey. As these experiences are more vast and mystical than simple words can encompass, art is a wonderful way to support integration.
- Invite them to journal about their experience. What transmissions did they receive? What epiphanies did they have? What was challenging about the experience? What wisdom do they want to bring forth with them?
- Give them space to talk through the journey in psychotherapy. As they do, reflect what they say, and ask them what they notice in their body. Support them in anchoring into this experience with thoughtful inquiries, like "How was that for you to experience …?" or "What aspect of this was significant for you?"
- If images and themes emerged, you can offer to do a more formal integration session using the same principles as working with a dream. The client would speak in the present moment from each element of the journey and become the full landscape of the experience.
- Refer them to an integration circle. Talking with other participants of psychedelic assisted therapy helps them to recognize the universal nature of the journey. Similarly, giving voice to this sacred experience in community expands and extends the experience.

Spiritual Emergency

Non-ordinary states are typically temporary experiences accessed during meditation, hypnosis, breathwork, psychedelics, or REM sleep. After we experience a non-ordinary state, it is helpful to integrate the experience into our ordinary awareness so that our ego can bring forth this new wisdom into our everyday lives and support us in our spiritual development. When a person has a sudden spiritual experience that dissolves their ego, their ordinary way of perceiving reality vanishes, and they can feel extremely disoriented. Because our ego helps us to navigate everyday life, without it we feel lost. As hyper-identification with thought-based reality disappears, so do identity, goals, values, and belief systems. The abrupt and unexpected nature of opening to a different reality can make it challenging to process, causing a psychospiritual crisis, known as a *spiritual emergency* (Grof & Grof, 1989).

While the experience of transcending the ego can be powerful and empowering, it can also be terrifying, messy, and painful. Features of psychosis, such as mania, insomnia, voices, visions, and emotional disturbances, are common, and clients can become increasingly unstable and afraid of being hospitalized. Through the colonized lens of the medical model, symptoms that accompany a spiritual emergency are commonly pathologized. While some people may find reassurance through suppressive techniques and hospitalization, this can be a very disempowering and traumatizing experience for many who experience a spiritual emergency.

As an acute presentation associated with a spiritual experience, rather than psychotic illness, this experience can be honored as a transition to growth. When handled with awareness, sensitivity, and care, a client can integrate this expansion into a new stage in their development, where they embody True Self awareness as a stage of consciousness, rather than a state. Although this is a highly spiritual experience that is, by definition, a non-ordinary state, it can be quite confusing to navigate on one's own. Through a nonviolent and integrative approach, we can honor the client's innate movement toward health as they find their way through the intensity and uncertainty of their experience.

Along with hyper-arousal of the nervous system, this expanded state of consciousness dissolves one's boundaries, where there is no sense of a separate self typically provided by the ego. There is also a sense of metaphysical uncertainty, where the client is unsure if they have a psychic intuition or are afraid and irrational. Depersonalization is also common, where a client feels as though they are watching themselves as if in a movie or a dream. By trusting our client's wholeness and organismic self-regulation, we offer them a safe place to find their way through the disorientation and into contact with themselves.

The balance of differentiating from the ego while still being functional in the world is one that many spiritual seekers grapple with. In cases of spiritual emergencies, cultivating practical and tangible habits for integration can allow a client to bring forth their true nature into the earthly realms. As they discover who they are now after the crisis of transformation, this experience can unfold into a deeply sacred and profound spiritual awakening. Once they have unlearned everything the ego thought was true, they get to rediscover how to trust themselves and engage with the environment in new and innovative ways.

Lessons from the Therapy Room

With clients, I only do dream work if they come to a session with a dream that they feel disturbed by or cannot make sense of. One such client came to a session telling me that she had had a dream where she was covered in feces. I asked her if she wanted to work with the dream, and she enthusiastically agreed.

First, she talked through the dream from her perspective: "I'm walking into a workshop with a group of participants. The workshop leader is telling us all to poop. I'm not sure why she wants us to do this, but I do it. Then I notice that everyone else is clean, and I am covered in shit. I try to hide it, but I smell so bad that it's obvious that I'm covered in shit. Everybody is looking at me wondering and disgusted by the smell."

As I listened, I heard various symbols: A workshop leader, workshop participants, feces, and the workshop facility.

Next, I invited her to become the workshop participants. As she talked through the dream again from this perspective, she became the participants who could do the activity properly and were disgusted by her dirtiness.

Then, she became the workshop leader, who told everyone to poop and eliminate their feces in the presence of everyone else. As the leader, she was confused about why the client was unable to do the activity properly, but she also ignored the client and didn't try to help her.

Next, she became the feces. "I'm shit. I'm all over (the client's) body. I won't get off of her. (The client) seems really upset that I'm here and she's trying to hide me. She doesn't want anybody else to see me, but I'm so stinky that everybody is looking."

She then became the workshop space. "There are people inside me who are here to learn and grow at this workshop. They are pooping, but one person is covered in poop. I see that she's ashamed and trying to hide, but nobody is helping her. She's with the group, but she feels all alone …."

Lastly, she talked through the dream again, from her perspective, as she wanted the dream to unfold, not wanting to see these different perspectives: "I'm walking into a workshop with other people. I feel separate from them but we are all here together. The workshop leader tells us to poop. We all poop, but everybody else is clean afterwards, and I'm covered in shit. I feel embarrassed, but I ask for help. Everyone comes over and helps to clean me."

The tender and beautiful landscape of this dream enabled my client to work through familiar themes in her life about not being enough, feeling alone in her suffering, and wanting to connect with others. The honesty and the purity of this dream allowed her to move through shame and see the importance of reaching out and asking for help.

Exercise: Dream Work Journaling

Choose a dream to journal about, and grab a piece of paper.

Step 1) Write your dream out as you remember it, as if it were happening right now. Make a note of how you feel as you do this.

Step 2) Underline or make a note of three or four different symbols or characters in the dream that stand out to you.

Step 3) Write out the dream from the perspective of the other symbols, noting how you feel as you do this. Repeat this until you have become all the symbols, including the landscape or structure you are on/in.

Step 4) Write out the dream again from your perspective, in the present moment, as if it were currently happening. Except this time, write the dream in the way you want it to unfold and resolve.

Step 5) Make a note of how this experience was for you.

References

Aixala, M. (2020). *Developing integration of visionary experiences: A future without integration.* Synergetic Press.

Aixala, M., & Bouso, J. C. (2022). *Psychedelic integration: Psychotherapy for non-ordinary states of consciousness.* Synergetic Press.

Barker, M. J., & Iantaffi, A. (2019). *Life isn't binary: On being both, beyond, and in-between.* Kingsley Publishers.

Beck, A. T. (2002). Cognitive patterns in dreams and daydreams. *Journal of Cognitive Psychotherapy, 16*(1), 23.

Blumberg, M. S., Lesku, J. A., Libourel, P. A., Schmidt, M. H., & Rattenborg, N. C. (2020). What is REM sleep? *Current Biology, 30*(1), R38–R49.

Bruhn, J. G., De Smet, P. A., El-Seedi, H. R., & Beck, O. (2002). Mescaline use for 5700 years. *Lancet, 359*(9320), 1866.

Fincham, G. W., Strauss, C., Montero-Marin, J., & Cavanagh, K. (2023). Effect of breathwork on stress and mental health: A meta-analysis of randomised-controlled trials. *Scientific Reports, 13*(432), 2045–2322.

Frecska, E. (2007). Therapeutic guidelines: Dangers and contra-indications in therapeutic applications of hallucinogens. In M. J. Winkelman & T. B. Roberts (Eds.), *Psychedelic medicine: New evidence for hallucinogenic substances as treatments* (pp. 69–95). Praeger Publishers.

Freud, S. (2010). *Interpretation of dreams: The complete and definitive text.* Basic Books.

Gorman, I., Nielson, E. M., Molinar, A., Cassidy, K., & Sabbagh, J. (2021). Psychedelic harm reduction and integration: A transtheoretical model for clinical practice. *Front Psychology, 12*, 645246.

Grof, S., & Grof, C. (1989). *Spiritual emergency: When personal transformation becomes a crisis* (1st ed.). TarcherPerigee.

Jung, C. (1909). *The analysis of dreams.* Newcomb Livraria Press.

Montes, C., & Penzenstadler, B. (2023). *Improved wellbeing and resilience via breathwork interventions for computer workers.* Chalmers University of Technology.

Mortaheb, S., Fort, L. D, Mason, N. L., Mallaroni, P., Ramaekers, J. G., & Demertzi, A. (2024). Dynamic functional hyperconnectivity after psilocybin intake is primarily associated with oceanic boundlessness. *Biological Psychiatry: Cognitive Neuroscience and Neuroimaging, 9*(7), 681–692.

Orr, L. (2013). *Haidakhan babaji speaks.* Hara Press.

Parrott, A. (2014). The potential dangers of using MDMA for psychotherapy. *The Journal of Psychoactive Drugs, 46*(1), 37–43.

Peever, J., & Fuller, P. M. (2017). The biology of REM sleep. *Current Biology, 27*(22), R1237–R1248.

Perls, F. (1992). *Gestalt therapy verbatim* (2nd Rev. ed.). The Gestalt Journal Press.

Strong, C. E., & Kabbaj, M. (2018). On the safety of repeated ketamine infusions for the treatment of depression: Effects of sex and developmental periods. Nurobiol Stress, 9, 166–175.

Szigeti, B., & Heifets, B. (2024). Expectancy Effects in Psychedelic Trials. *Biological Psychiatry: Cognitive Neuroscience and Neuroimaging, 9*(5), 512–521.

Ziff, S., Stern, B., Lewis, G., Majeed, M., & Gorantla, V. R. (2022). Analysis of psilocybin-assisted therapy in medicine: A narrative review. *Cureus, 14*(2), e21944.

Spiritual Self-Care

Chapter 16

The calling to be an awakened therapist is unique in that the potential for what unfolds in our therapeutic container is synergistic with our spiritual health. Our presence either interrupts or supports our clients' ability to ignite their natural Source of healing. When we are under-resourced, identified with our thinking mind, and/or ignoring our own blind spots, we are unable to be a clear mirror of reflection. Over half of therapists experience burnout, and half of those therapists leave the profession after two years (Canady, 2023; Emery et al., 2012; McCormack et al., 2018). Although we do not need to be completely enlightened in order to do this work well, we do need to actively and regularly build our inner resources, differentiate from our mind, clear and tone our energy, and integrate our shadow in order to tend to our own well-being.

When we take good care of ourselves, our wakeful presence allows us to be fully and authentically engaged in the therapeutic process. It may seem as though bringing a high quality of presence into our work would lead to burnout. Burnout occurs when we *give our energy away* to our clients, when we try to *carry their burden*, and when we *energetically take them home* with us. In these moments, we ignore our somatic sensations, forget to breathe, and bypass our intuitive senses. Subsequently, we lack the inner spaciousness needed to do this work, and we end up processing clients' emotions for them.

Both within our work and in our personal life, the way we tend to our energy either inspires or interferes with our ability to hold space with such clear intention. When we work with clients from an awakened state, we trust that they have their own Source of energy within them, and we stay aligned with our own Source of energy. Noticing when we feel tension or contraction in our body, breathing up and down our midline, and honoring our intuitive sensitivities is not only a gift for the client—it is an act of energetic self-care. We deepen into our alignment as our clients discover their alignment, and synergistically, we both leave the session feeling more lit up about life.

DOI: 10.4324/9781003521969-19

Therapists' Contact Boundary Disturbances

The unconscious habits of our personality can create a murky container, where we disrupt contact and take on our clients' energy. Unknowingly, we become induced in our clients' inner world and collude with their patterns, making it harder to see them clearly or to be a clear mirror of reflection. We end up swimming in our clients' emotions and lose access to our higher consciousness. From our personality, our energy centers are more prone to hold our clients' experience, and we end up processing their emotions for them. Over time, engaging from our personality with their personality causes us to burn out and be less effective.

As we continue to heal and transform, our own contact disruptions are less likely to impede and interrupt our clients' process and innate movement toward health. When we are in full contact, we are able to be fully present and authentically engaged in the therapeutic relationship. From this place, we witness and reflect our clients with clarity. Our intuitive senses are heightened, and we are able to utilize intuitive transmissions in a way that maintains contact with the client. All of the insight gathered, felt, and sensed in a therapeutic container that is characterized by awareness and contact is information about the client's inner world that we can use to support their transformation.

When we meet our clients at the contact boundary, our effort becomes more efficient, and our interventions become more effective. From a contactful place, we actually do quite a lot by doing very little. The strategies that a client uses to avoid contact become more apparent when we are fully present at the sacred boundary. They become more aware through our reflection, and we support them as they find their way back into presence and into contact with their true nature.

Here are some ways our own contact boundary disturbances might show up in a session and how to mitigate these tendencies:

♦ When you turn away from your somatic experience as you hold space, your tendency to *deflect* impedes your presence. Similarly, when you turn away from your intuitive wisdom, you avoid confronting incongruence in the client.
  ○ The best way to take care of yourself in real time during a session is to breathe. Breathing the breath of self-care reminds clients to breathe, too. This helps you to create a more spacious container as you co-regulate.
  ○ When habits of your personality cause you to avoid naming the implicit, you keep yourself from being in full contact. Honoring your clear seeing and offering an accurate reflection of how the client seems is a movement of turning towards what's here as opposed to deflecting.
♦ When you bring your *introjections* into a session, you see your clients through the veil of your own cultural lens and acquired ideas. Assuming you know what a client means when they use certain words is one way your introjections can become imbued in a session.
  ○ Awareness of your own introjected ideas and values is essential to guiding a session contactfully. Assume nothing when holding space. Be curious about what a client wants for themselves and what they mean when they use certain

language. Even simple words can be used in different ways: Anxious can mean eager or scared; uncertain can mean confused or open to possibilities; frustrated can mean angry or thwarted.

♦ *Projections* occur in a session with countertransference, where your client unconsciously reminds you of someone in your personal life. Denying your own impulse to rescue them or judge them, you see them through the lens of your own wounding.

    ○ Actively look at your own blind spots and integrate your shadow to mitigate projections and countertransference. Projections aren't wrong—they are simply a sense within yourself pointed in the wrong direction. Countertransference isn't bad; it is information for you to be curious about.

    ○ While these blind spots must be worked out in your own therapy or supervision, there is a simple way to mitigate them in real time: Use language where you *own your experience*. Hold your perspective loosely, then see what is true for the client. Using the language of ownership keeps the container clean and honors this work as deeply collaborative.

♦ *Retroflections* occur when you become hard on yourself to know better or do better for your clients. The trap of this is thinking that if you did better, then they could do better.

    ○ Welcome your clients as they are, and welcome yourself as you are. Each day offers ongoing learning opportunities, and to have a growth-oriented mindset means that you accept yourself as you currently are. After each session, contemplating what you would have done differently can be a useful way to continue to evolve in your skills.

♦ When you hold space from a state of *confluence*, a session can feel confusing and murky. You can easily get induced into the client's inner experience, and you can get hooked into being the rescuer. This is a quick road to burnout.

    ○ One of the most effective real-time tools for overcoming therapeutic confluence is reflective listening. However, when you reflect, energetically give the client their words back to them. This reinforces that this is what they think and feel, and not necessarily what you think and feel. It cleans the therapeutic container and strengthens the therapeutic boundary.

Surrendering to the Sacred

When our personality guides our therapy sessions, we play the role of the expert and think we need to have all of the answers for our clients. Working hard to fix our clients or trying to change them in any way is exhausting. Because this is their work to do, expending our energy to do the work for them is depleting. Even when we have this knowledge and intend to hold a truly transpersonal container, we can still unconsciously collude with the client's perceived helplessness and try to rescue them from their suffering.

Moving beyond the personal realm of the ordinary mind and holding a container that is truly transpersonal, we trust that our client's soul knows what they need to heal. Allowing Spirit to be our co-therapist, we trust that our client's awareness and innate wisdom can guide them in their healing. Respecting our clients enough to honor their inherent wisdom, their timing, and their sovereign choice, we meet them at the altar of their transformation.

This work is holy. Sitting with clients in the depths of their uncertainty, pain, and longing is a sacred honor. To do this work, we must be congruent within ourselves as we hold space. Our thoughts, words, and actions must align with the truth of who we are as we let go of any preconceived notion of our ego identity. When the container we hold is set through our most awake and conscious Self, the energy of Divine Spirit guides what unfolds. Our idea of our *self* recedes, and we become a vessel to encounter the sacred in therapy.

Because the ordinary mind can convince us that we need to do more or work harder, daily practices that reinforce our commitment to the sacred realms of healing can be helpful. Pausing for devotional prayer every morning and/or before each client is a wonderful way to remind our ego that Divine Spirit is guiding the work that unfolds in a session. Intentionally inviting the transpersonal realms of spirituality to be at the center of our work, we surrender deeply to the relational meditation that is gestalt therapy.

Stages of Skill Acquisition

Learning to stay awake and aware with clients is an ongoing endeavor. Doing this while also learning a new framework and new interventions can feel daunting. The beauty of this work is that it evolves as we evolve. Every time we shift and repair internally, the way we meet our clients is different.

When we try to do this work perfectly, our idea of perfect impedes our authentic engagement and intuitive transmissions. The more experience we have with the dialogic relationship, the more we trust that our presence and witness are powerful. The more we open into the field of awareness, the more intuitive wisdom can guide the therapeutic process.

Practice and awareness are integral to the process of acquiring new skills. As we move from unaware and effortful to aware and easeful, understanding the levels of competence can support our own self-compassion and growth mindset.

The stages described here are adapted from *The Four Stages of Competence* (Broadwell, 1969):

Stage 1: Unconsciously incompetent: This is when you are unaware of the patterns of thinking and behaving that inhibit your ability to stay in contact.

Stage 2: Consciously incompetent: This is when you develop the awareness of your patterns, but you are not sure how to do something differently.

Stage 3: Consciously competent: This is when you use your conscious choice to do something different and truer.

Stage 4: Unconsciously competent: This is when you have the capacity to do the different, truer thing without needing to think about doing it. It's integrated into your way of being.

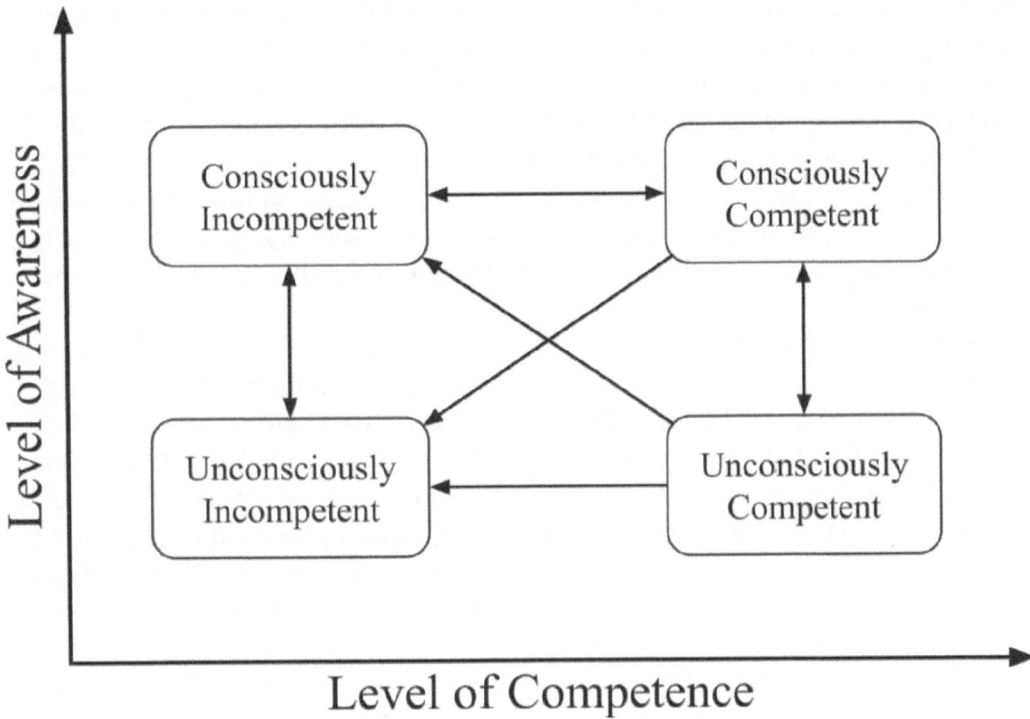

Figure 16.1 Skill Acquisition (Kwiker, 2023, p. 332)

These stages are not linear. As we move through cycles of wakefulness and forgetfulness, we find ourselves at different points in this stage model (Figure 16.1).

Tending to Your Energy

Because our own inner clarity and spaciousness are needed for this deep level of work, taking care of our energy is paramount. All of us carry around emotional energy pollution (EEP) in our energy body. Even when we actively care for our own well-being, the daily experiences of humanity—driving, technology, relational interactions, and so on—can cause the emotional residue of our experiences to accumulate in our energy body. When we forget to clear our own EEP, we eventually have less bandwidth to hold space for our clients.

Aside from holding an energetically clean container, our own commitment to daily practices can support the clarity of our energy. As we explored in an earlier chapter, there are five ways to move energy: 1) *awareness*, 2) *breath*, 3) *sound*, 4) *touch*, and 5) *movement*. When we feel depleted or stuck in our energy body, these five resources are always freely accessible.

Nature holds the remedy to imbalances caused by burnout. By honoring the four sacred elements, our energetic self-care is in rhythm with the natural world. The following are significant resources for energetic self-care:

- **Water:** The sacred element of water is connected to emotions, wisdom, and flow. When you submerge your chakras in water, your energy body feels held in such a way that you can surrender. You clear away the emotional energy you're holding, and your energy centers can reset. When you're feeling heavy with emotion, soaking in water can be extremely resourceful.
  - Taking an hour-long bath once a week can anchor you into the lived experience of opening to the flow of water. Natural water sources, such as hot springs, lakes, and oceans, are also amazing resources for this deeply clarifying experience.
- **Fire:** The sacred element of fire can transmute anger and depression. It can ignite inspiration and passion, and it can support your transmutation of stuck energy.
  - Sitting by a wood-burning fire for at least an hour is ideal to access the potency of this sacred element. Candles and gas fireplaces can also be a wonderful way to bring this element into your consciousness to support your inner balance.
- **Earth:** The sacred element of earth can offer grounding and support embodiment. When connected to the earth, you are fully present in the here and now. Earth relates to your work—your career and service, as well as washing dishes and doing laundry.
  - Eating foods that grow in the earth (root vegetables), digging in the earth, or standing barefoot on the earth can anchor you into the grounding resource of the earth element. Likewise, plant medicine can also be considered the earth element.
- **Air:** The sacred element of air can clarify your energy body, move anxiety, and remind you what it feels like to be alive and vital. Air relates to your intellectual state, and when you honor this element, you can calm your mind and access deep presence.
  - Breathwork is the sacred and transpersonal practice of conscious breathing practices. Connected breathing (in and out of the nose, without stopping at the top or the bottom of the breath) can activate the self-cleaning mechanism of the breath and reset the nervous system (Goldman, 2017). Standing in the wind, dancing, and running can also access the sacred element of air.

While each element is potent in and of itself, using all four elements together at one time can amplify their potency and bring us back into alignment. The rhythm of nature and its elements offer the remedies needed from living in an unwell society. To embody our wholeness is to disengage from the systems that tell us we are broken and to align with our true nature. From this place, our presence on the planet contributes to the well-being of all beings. We become the safety, health, love, and abundance that we long for, and the world is forever changed.

Lessons from the Therapy Room

When I was a child in the 80s, the outgoing message on our answering machine ended with my mom saying, "And as always, remember to breathe. Ahhhhhh." Although I was mortified at the time, I now recognize the beauty and the gift of this sweet reminder. My mom was a wise healer and a breathwork teacher. Individual and group breathwork sessions happened in my home daily. As I watched cartoons in my living room, I could hear my mom's clients moving through trauma and returning to their bliss body in the room next to me.

I started practicing breathwork and Transcendental Meditation at a very young age, so I learned early on how non-ordinary states of consciousness could be a mystical resource on this journey of life. When I became a therapist, though, I was unaware of how important breathwork and other energy practices would be for my self-care. In the newness of holding space for clients, I would think about clients and what had happened in their sessions for several days, oftentimes losing sleep as I mulled over how to help them. My sense of self became consumed by my work, and I found myself processing their emotions and thoughts during my leisure time.

My body felt dense, my soul felt tired, and my mind would fantasize about becoming an interior designer. I realized that if I were to be a good therapist, I needed to find a way to tend to my own energy in real time as I held space, as well as after a day of work. I began working with my energy in sessions, moving through feelings of discomfort and stuckness along with my clients. I used my words and my awareness to give their energy back to them, and I would guide them in processing their own emotions. This helped tremendously.

In my own time, I would shower or bathe after each day of work, allowing the water to wash away the emotional energy pollution. I also created practices to clear my energy body with awareness, intention, breath, movement, sound, and touch. The most profound tool in my self-care, however, was found when I reconnected with breathwork. It had been at least 15 years since I had practiced conscious connected breathing, and when I found myself in a private session practicing again, I felt like I was home. After breathing, I felt inspired, excited, and honored to serve my clients on their journey. I felt spacious and free, and I could bring this liberation with me into my work.

The wisdom of the breath has the power to bring me back into balance with such ease and grace. All of the sacred elements are my teachers and guides, and I am so grateful for the resources of air, fire, earth, and water.

I also have three daily devotional practices that I do in the morning, in the shower, and at night:

♦ **Morning ritual:** In the morning, I sit in meditation and align with Divine Spirit. Then, I ask for guidance in bringing more consciousness into all my thoughts, words, and actions. I say aloud, "Divine Spirit, I ask that Your wisdom, consciousness, love, and truth be at the center of everything I think, everything I say, everything I do, and all that I Am. Please guide my actions and make clear the way. I live this life to serve You." Being intentional about where I am living from is the most important component of my morning ritual.

♦ **Energy clearing in the shower:** Every day when I take a shower, I do an energy clearing practice where I set my boundaries. I begin by asking my spirit guides for help clearing my energy. I say aloud, "I ask all of my guides, helpers, fairies, and angels to identify, locate, and remove any energy living in my system that does not originate with me and is not mine to process. I ask that it be returned to its proper source immediately." Then, I picture this in my mind's eye when I say, "Other people's judgments, emotions, projections, and so on ... may it be cleared from my system immediately." If there is a specific person I can feel in my energetic space, I say their name and give them their energy back.

- Next, I set my energetic boundary by tapping my sternum with the fingertips of my right hand while I hold my left hand in front of me like a stop sign. From the core of my being, I energetically push out and say, "Any time others think of me, may it bounce off of my energetic boundary and they get redirected to the Source that Beats their Heart. When I think of others, may it bounce off of their energetic boundary and I get redirected to the Source that Beats my Heart. May we all feel more aligned for having come into one another's sphere."

♦ **Evening practice:** At night, I close my day by sitting in meditation and contemplating forgiveness. With my physical eyes closed, I look back over my day to remember anyone I felt harmed me and anyone I might have harmed. I say aloud, "May I forgive those who have offended me today, either knowingly or unknowingly. And may I ask for forgiveness from those whom I offended today, either knowingly or unknowingly." Using my breath and awareness, I clean up the day's energetic interactions.

Exercise: Self-Energy Clearing

1. Begin by attuning to your alignment with the Source that Beats Your Heart. You may want to speak this invocation aloud: "I ask that part of myself that knows how to do it to align with the Source that beats my heart."
2. Use your hands, breath, and awareness to clear your energetic space.
3. Invite support from alternate dimensions to fully clear your energy body: "I ask all my helpers and guides to identify, locate, and remove any energy living in my system that does not belong to me and give it back to its proper source immediately."
4. If there is a specific encounter or person that you feel being held in your energy body, specify that: "I give back any judgments, projections, or emotions that belong to (person's name)."
5. Now, amend any place where you have leaked or projected energy: "I take back any energy that I have given away. I take back my judgments, projections, emotions, and power."
6. Stay in silence with your breath as your energy continues to clear.
7. If there are ongoing relational challenges with a specific person, cultivate relational alignment: "I ask that any time (this person) thinks about me, it bounces off my energetic boundary and gets redirected back to the Source that beats their heart. And any time I think of them, I ask that I get redirected to the Source that beats my heart."
8. Lastly, bring this with you into your life: "I ask that this go on in all directions of space and time until complete."

Final Thoughts and Wishes

Therapists tend to hold a high bar for themselves. Wanting to do the best for our clients, we can often wonder if we know enough to guide clients through the nuanced terrain of their inner world. Uncertain if awareness and presence are enough, we wonder if we are healed enough to help others.

The way we are with anything is the way we are with everything. If we treat ourselves as an object—an expert who needs to know everything and be all the way healed—we, in turn, objectify our clients. If we treat ourselves as a dynamic living being, we treat our clients as dynamic living beings. To treat ourselves as a sacred vessel reflects outwardly to the way we treat our clients. If we treat every aspect of life as sacred, every moment with our clients is a sacred honor.

Instead of doubting our knowledge and capacity, let us inquire how our path of healing and ongoing learning can serve our clients. As we continue on our own personal journey, we also walk with our clients, metaphorically holding their hand as they find their way back to their deepest and truest Self. Without personalizing our clients' experience, we can allow their souls to discover what is needed for deep repair and healing. Together, we return to the vibration of true nature over and over again, until our increased state of consciousness becomes an increased stage of consciousness.

In the decades that I have been doing this work, my love of humanity is strengthened every time I sit with a client. The sacred nature of the human condition still motivates me to keep showing up. Over the years, I have learned that when I tend to myself and my clients with reverence, this reverence guides my every breath, every word, and every therapeutic intervention with my clients and my students. Deep within my soul, I know that I am only a healer to the degree that my presence reminds others that they are already whole. For me, this is what makes the therapeutic container a sacred vessel of transformation.

I thank you, deeply, for your dedication to your craft and your clients. I thank you for your commitment to your own consciousness and healing. And I thank you for being a catalyst for the greater healing of the planet. There is so much suffering in this world, and your presence on this planet forever impacts the greater collective. I honor you as you continue to awaken to the therapist you were born to be.

References

Broadwell, M. M. (1969). *Teaching for learning (XVI)*. The Gospel Guardian.
Canady, V. (2023). More than half of mental health therapists experience burnout. *Mental health Weekly*, 33(39): 5–6.

Emery, S., Wade, T., & McLean, S. (2009). *Associations among therapist beliefs, personal resources and burnout in clinical psychologists. Behaviour Change, 26*(2), 83–96.

Goldman, B. (2017). Study shows how slow breathing induces tranquility. Stanford Medicine, News Center.

Kwiker, H. (2022). *Align: Living and loving from the true self.* Mantra Books.

McCormack, H. M., Macintyre, T. E., O'Shea, D, Herring, M. P., & Campbell, M. J. (2018). The prevalence and cause(s) of burnout among applied psychologists: a systematic review. *Fronteirs in Psychology, 9*(1897), https://pmc.ncbi.nlm.nih.gov/articles/PMC6198075/#abstract1.

Workbook

Chapter 17, "Workbook," offers clear and effective exercises to implement the concepts of *The Awakened Therapist*. In this chapter, you will learn how to stay in contact with yourself as you lead a session, how to explore the sacred boundary in the therapeutic container, how to explore subtle energy and honor somatic intelligence, and how to be culturally reflexive. Exercises to explore identifying and working with each of the five contact boundary disturbances are provided, as well as practicing how to map a client's inner world. There are exercises to support you in creating various gestalt experiments and exploring your own ideas regarding transpersonal parts work and psychedelic assisted therapy. From staying seated in one's self, to working with subtle energy, to exploring the gestalt therapeutic cycle, these worksheets support deepening understanding of this work.

Activity 1: Self-Check-In Before a Session

Before we step into a session, we must establish a baseline of our state of being. This helps us to stay connected to ourselves, which is paramount to preventing unconscious processing of our clients' emotions for them. This practice also prevents burnout.

Close your eyes, and notice how it feels to be you in this moment. Take a few breaths, and scan your inner world to get a baseline of how you feel right now.

On a scale of one to ten, rate the following.

1 is the most tension and cloudiness, and 10 is the most clear and open.

Mind: 1   2   3   4   5   6   7   8   9   10

Body: 1   2   3   4   5   6   7   8   9   10

Emotions: 1   2   3   4   5   6   7   8   9   10

Energy: 1 2   3   4   5   6   7   8   9   10

DOI: 10.4324/9781003521969-20

Vitality: 1 2   3   4   5   6   7   8   9   10

Awareness: 1   2   3   4   5   6   7   8   9   10

Mantra: This is me. This is mine. I tend to myself in service of being a clear mirror, and I allow my client to process their own emotions.

Repeat as needed to remind yourself of the sacred boundary.

Activity 2: Exploring the Sacred Boundary

The sacred boundary is the point in which you contact your client without going over into their space. This means that your thoughts, your desires, your perceptions, and your energy are yours to own. Similarly, the client's thoughts, desires, perceptions, and energy are theirs to become aware of and process as their own.

In a single session, the mind tracks various details, while higher consciousness explores the awareness field. If we consider percentages of our attention, about 60% is on the client, 20% is on our inner experience, and 20% is on the space between, the I–Thou relationship.

Recall a recent session with a client. Put all of your attention on your inner experience during that session. What narratives did you have about the client? How did you feel while sitting with them? In Figure 17.1, write the insights you discovered in the therapist circle.

Repeat the process for the client circle. How did they seem during the session? What was the essence of their feelings and narratives? Write your observations in the client circle.

Repeat the process again for the I–Thou relationship. What was the quality of contact between you and the client? What was the energy like in the "we" space?

Repeat the process for the therapeutic container. How did the container seem to you? Clear? Murky? Something else?

Finally, try bringing attention to all areas simultaneously. What insights can you gather?

Activity 3: Exploring Subtle Awareness

Subtle awareness reveals the blocks and movements of a client's energy body. When we explore subtle awareness, we bring attunement to the client's energy in a pure and unfiltered way.

Try to recall a past experience when you walked into a place that stored a lot of emotional energy pollution (EEP). The place may have been a dive bar or even a retreat center with shadowy leadership. In the space below, journal about this experience:

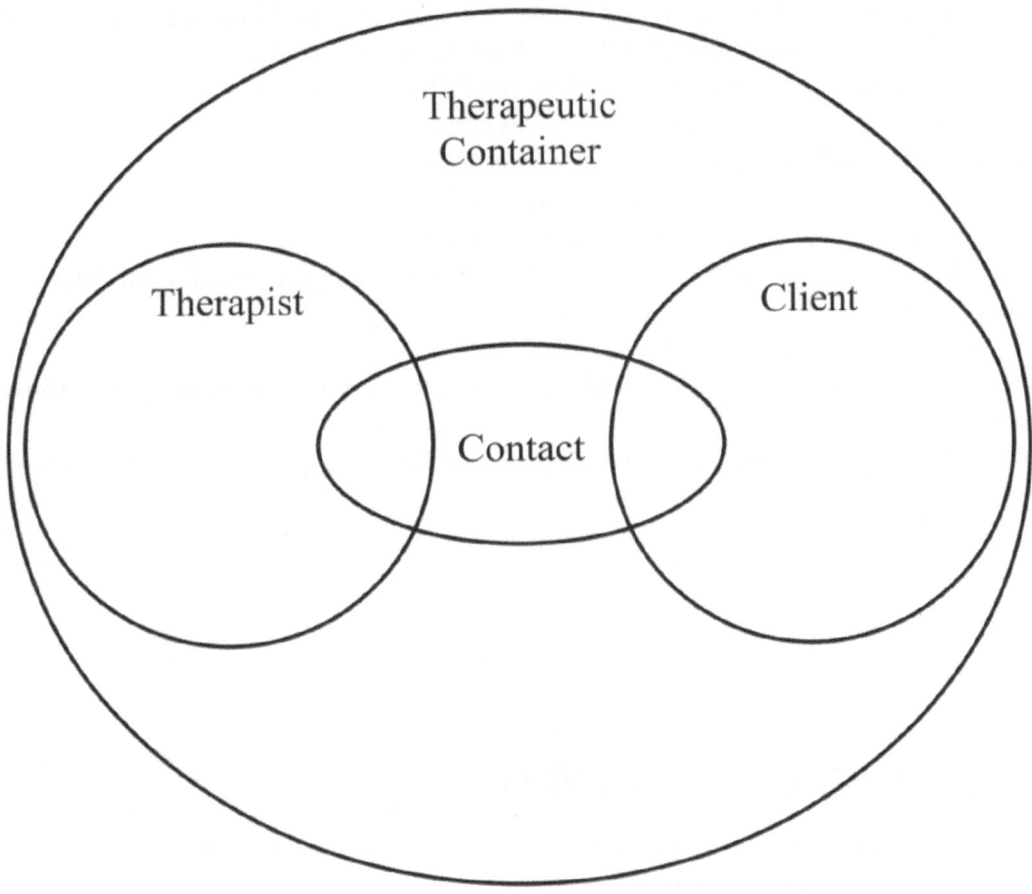

Figure 17.1 Therapeutic Container

What did this EEP look like?

What did you sense in your body?

How did the space seem to you?

Now, recall a walked-into space that felt clear and sparkly. The place may have been a yoga studio or the home of a friend who tends to the EEP. In the space below, journal about this experience:

What did the clarity look like?

What did you sense in your body?

How did the space seem to you?

These principles of exploring subtle energy also apply to human beings. When the illusions of our mind are clear, we can see where EEP is being stored, when it moves, and when it is clear.

Activity 4: Opening to Somatic Intelligence

Turning away from our somatic intelligence is the result of deflection. By practicing opening up to somatic intelligence, we can quiet the mind and come into direct experience. From this presence, hearing the body's messages becomes quite accessible. There is no need to interpret or figure out the body's messages. It will tell you when you listen.

Part 1: In a journal, write your answers to the following inquiries:

Describe one sensation your body is feeling right now.

Describe the shape, size, and color of the sensation.

If this sensation had a voice, what would it say?

What does this sensation need from you right now?

Part 2: Think of a client you recently sat with for a session, and write your answers to the following inquiries:

How did you feel when you sat with this client?

In the most neutral language, without narratives, what word or words get to the essence of this feeling?

If you were not personalizing this feeling, how would you guess this relates to the client's inner experience?

Activity 5: Cultural Reflexivity

Much of our internalized racism and racialized trauma lives in the body. Use this space to journal and answer the following questions:

What sensations do you experience in your body when you encounter a person with a different racial identity? If possible, consider an encounter with a client.

What sensations do you experience when you reflect on your body's reaction to racial differences?

What narratives do notice your mind creating about yourself? About the other person?

What narratives do you create about the values of the other person's culture?

What values do you think you may share with them?

Activity 6: Identifying Deflection

Find a practice client to record a session with. If this is not accessible to you, then think of a client you have worked with. Review the recording of the session, and write down how they express their deflection. Remember that deflection is the impulse to turn away from discomfort in oneself and in the environment (Figure 17.2). For example, you might observe your client laughing when they say they feel angry.

What thoughts or behaviors emerge in this client when they deflect?

How does their deflection serve them?

How might you support their increasing awareness of their tendency to deflect?

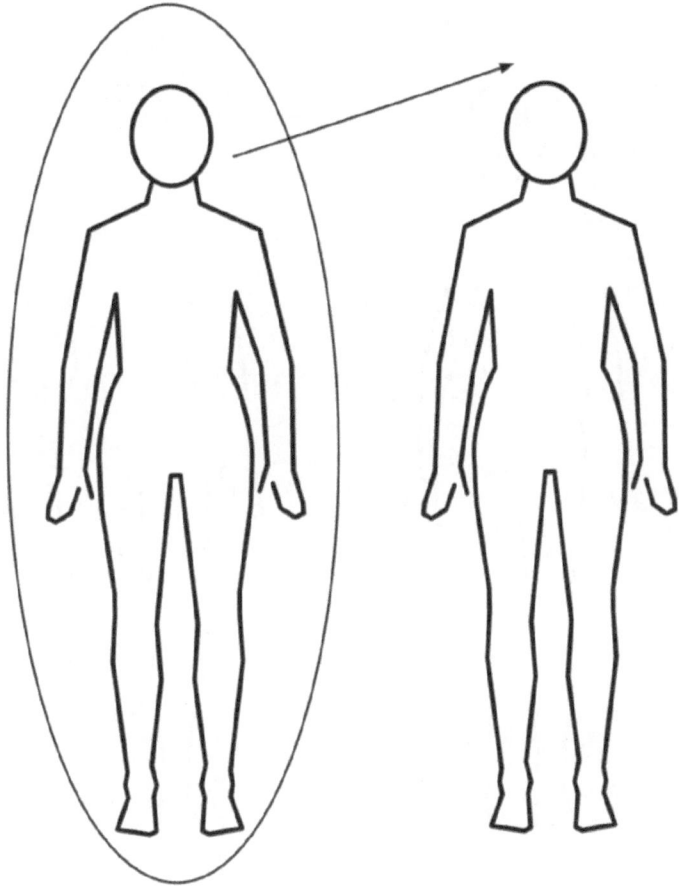

Figure 17.2 Deflection (Kwiker, 2022, p. 112)

Activity 7: Identifying Introjection

Find a practice client to record a session with. If this is not accessible to you, then think of a client you've worked with. Review the recording of the session, and write down how they express their introjection. Remember that introjections are undigested beliefs, values, and behaviors that are acquired from the environment and living in the client's personality (Figure 17.3).

What thoughts or themes emerge in this client that express an introjected value or belief?

What is the birthplace of (i.e. where did they acquire) their introjection?

How is the introjection expressed through their personality?

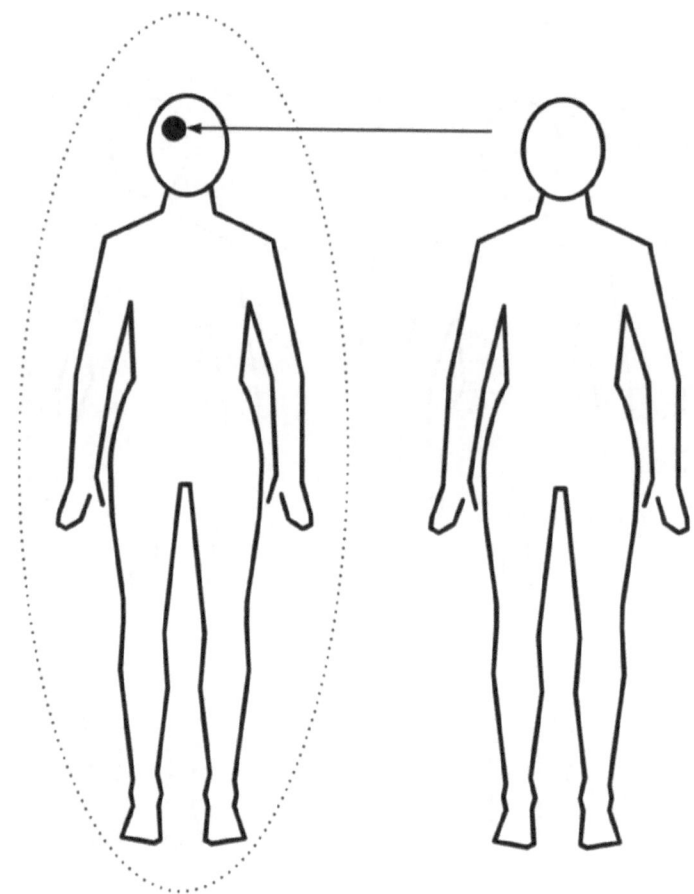

Figure 17.3 Introjection (Kwiker, 2022, p. 107)

Activity 8: Identifying Projection

Find a practice client to record a session with. If this is not accessible to you, then think of a client you work with. Review the recording of the session, and write down how they express their projections. Remember that projections are a mechanism for denying something within oneself and putting it onto the environment (Figure 17.4).

What narratives or themes of relationships emerge in this client that express projections?
What illusion are they projecting, and what truth does that reveal about them?
What are their projections about others mirroring back about them?
What reflection can you offer your client about what they are avoiding within themselves?

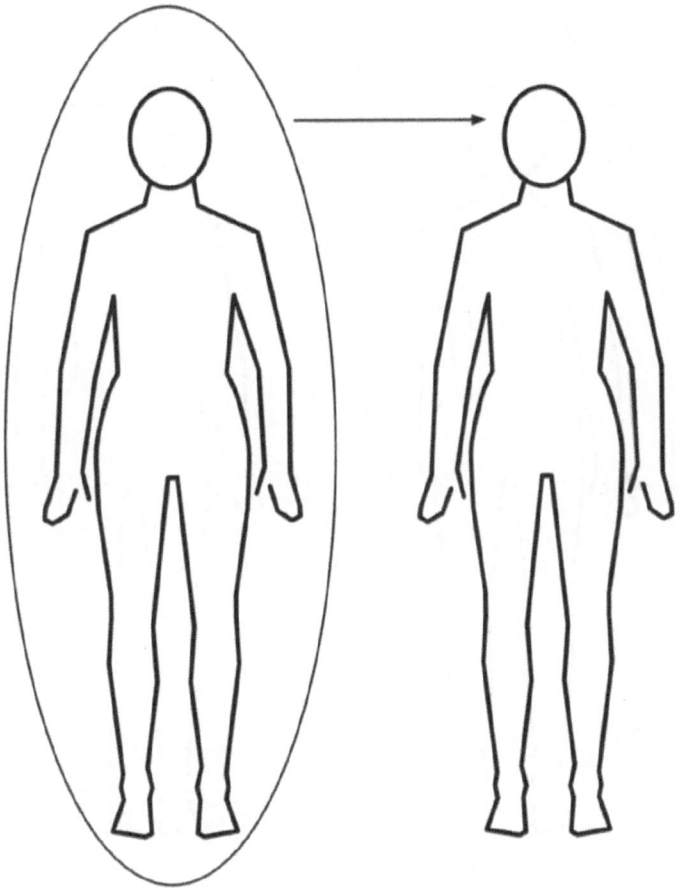

Figure 17.4 Projection (Kwiker, 2022, p. 108)

Activity 9: Identifying Retroflection

Find a practice client to record a session with. If this is not accessible to you, then think of a client you work with. Review the recording of the session, and write down how they express their retroflection.

   Retroflection: Putting on oneself what a person cannot say to people in their environment (Figure 17.5).

   What thoughts express that this client turned in on themselves what you think they would have likely wanted to say to their caregivers in childhood?

   What would you imagine this client would have wanted to say to their caregivers?

   How did that thought get turned against themselves?

   How could you support your client in having that idea redirected to its original source?

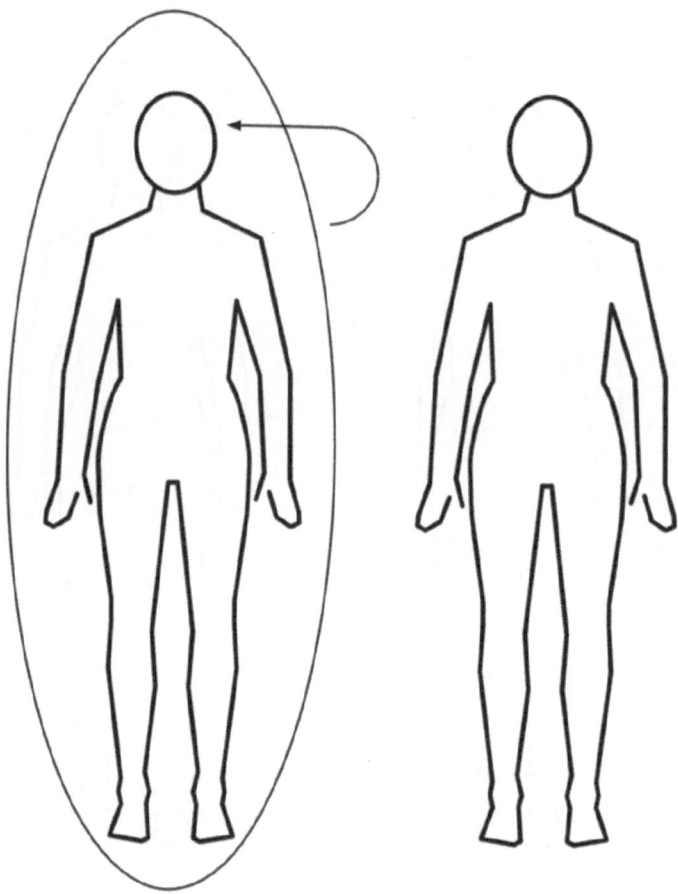

Figure 17.5 Retroflection (Kwiker, 2022, p. 111)

Activity 10: Identifying Confluence

Find a practice client to record a session with. If this is not accessible to you, then think of a client you have worked with. Review the recording of the session, and write down how they express their confluence. Remember that confluence is when a person lacks a sense of self separate from the environment, causing their sense of well-being to be dependent on others (Figure 17.6).

What thoughts or behaviors express the client's tendency to merge with others?

What environmental circumstance triggers the merging/confluence for your client?

What would their authentic expression be if not merging with others?

How can you support your client in unblending from the environment?

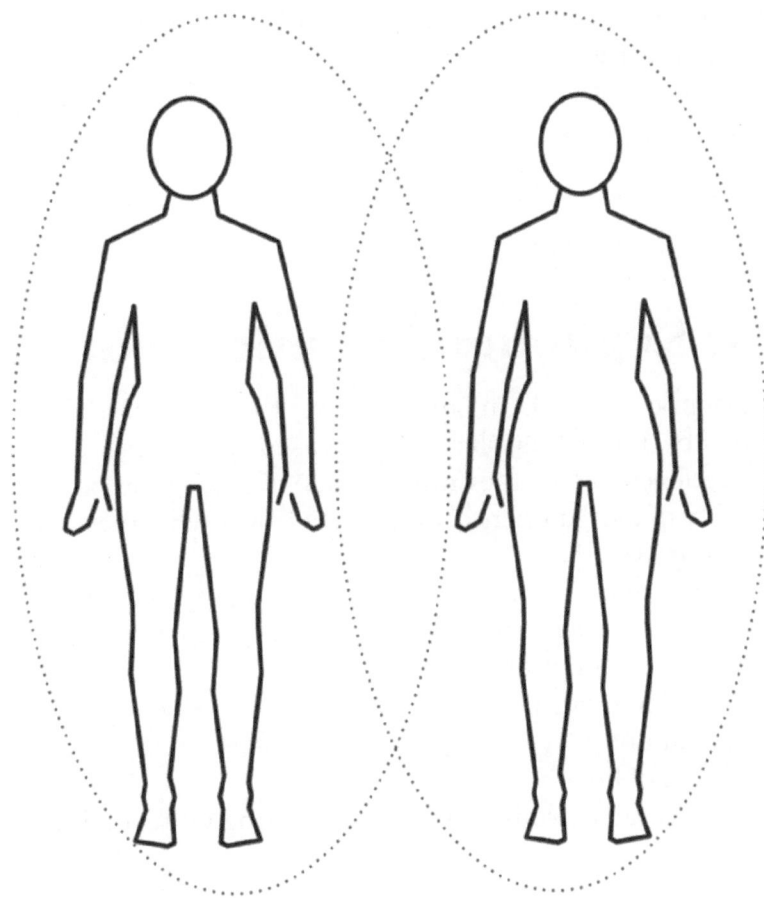

Figure 17.6 Confluence (Kwiker, 2022, p. 110)

Activity 11: Discovering the Map

Building on the work you did in activities 7–11, use the same recording or recollection of a client that you see regularly. Create a map of their inner world:

What are the primary misbeliefs and narratives that pull the attention of their ordinary mind?

How identified do they seem with their thought-based reality?

What are their biggest blind spots?

How do they relate to the sensations in their body?

What emotions do they get stuck in?

What is their relationship to their desire?

What is their relationship to their power?

What is their relationship to the present moment?

What is their relationship to the future?

How does their subtle energy body seem?

What polarity seems to pull them off center?

How do all of these threads come together into the formation of a Gestalt? What's the common thread between these landmarks?

Activity 12: Exploring Somatic Awareness

Somatic awareness supports clients in shifting from their thought-based reality into their awareness-based reality. From this place of increased awareness, a client can be in the actuality of their experience, even if they are in a state of dysregulation. By inviting the client to embody the actuality of the experience, they can discover what they need from themselves to regulate their nervous system.

Building on the work you did in activity 11, consider ways you can support your client with increasing their *somatic awareness*. What invitations might you offer?

Increasing awareness of sensations:

Increasing awareness of movement:

Exploring self-validation:

Increasing awareness of breath:

Which of these experiments would you consider trying with your client?

Activity 13: Identifying Polarities and Creating Two-Chair Experiments

Step 1: Identify a Polarity

A polarity consists of two seemingly opposing aspects of the client's inner world. The top-dog of the polarity is the loudest voice of a client's mind, and the under-dog is the deeper truth that they deny or resist.

Building on the work you did in activity 11, identify a top-dog and an under-dog voice.

What is the main theme of a client's narrative (top-dog)? What is their predominant strategy as they engage with their environment?

What do they resist within their narratives (under-dog)? What truth is pushed into their shadow?

Step 2: Design a Two-Chair Experiment

Experiments happen naturally and are co-created with the client in the present moment. However, as we learn to be creative in the therapeutic container, it can be useful to contemplate what experiments might work well with a given client. Remember, experiments are meant to increase awareness of where there was a previously unknown potential. Two-chair experiments are integrative, with the top-dog and the under-dog each in their own chair.

Considering the client you mapped out in activity 11, journal about what *two-chair experiments* you might want to explore.

Polarities present in the client:

Language the client has used that indicates these polarities:

How to unblend these polarities:

How to integrate these polarities:

Activity 14: Creating Shadow Work Experiments

Because the shadow inherently lives in a person's blind spot, shadow work can be extremely illuminating for a client. Aspects of themselves that they think make them unlovable can be illuminated with awareness and compassion. In a safe and non-judgmental container, a client can move through shame and integrate what they have disowned or rejected about themselves.

Think of the client you mapped out in activity 11. What shadow work experiments would you create with this client?

What do you see in their blind spot?

How does the client relate to their shadow?

What experiment might you suggest to increase awareness, learning, and self-compassion?

Activity 15: Creating Experiments to Complete Unfinished Business

Most of the constructs we work with in a session are the result of unfinished business. However, some sessions are more focused on specific memories the client has of unresolved experiences. These memories of past events are preventing the client from being fully present in the here and now.

Consider the client you mapped out in activity 11. What experiments would you create to support the completion of unfinished business?

What is the unfinished business you believe might be holding your client back?

What reparenting experiment might you try to help them resolve this unfinished business?

What empty chair experiment might you try?

What unique experiment might you create and try?

Activity 16: Creating Art Experiments

Artistic exploration can help clients to express their thoughts and feelings in deep and meaningful ways. Art can also help clients to access a part of the brain that holds memories beyond the logic of the thinking brain. Creating experiments with art offers imagery and expression that can illuminate the client's energetic holding patterns.

Consider the client you mapped out in activity 11. What creative art experiment might you try?

What experience, thought, memory, or behavior do you see holding the client back?

How might you invite the client to represent this in art?

What other art experiments could support this client in relating to their experience in deep and meaningful ways?

Activity 17: Transpersonal Parts Work

When learning about transpersonal parts work, it is common to be apprehensive about doing this work with clients. Remember that transpersonal parts work includes toxic elements introjected from the environment. These introjections do not need to be assimilated and can be cleared from the client's system. In the space below, journal about how you relate to transpersonal parts work.

How do you feel when you consider the concept of transpersonal parts work?

How do you feel when you consider applying transpersonal parts work with your clients?

How do you think you'll respond if this emerges in a therapeutic session?

How could you support yourself so you feel confident in guiding this deep work?

Activity 18: Psychedelic Integration

Because psychedelic assisted therapy (PAT) is a newer opportunity in the field of mental health, it's important to explore our relationship to psychedelics. Even if you do not participate in or advocate for PAT, you are affected. Similarly, even if you have tremendous practice and lineage with PAT, being conscious with your relationship with it is valuable.

Journal about how you relate to PAT.

What biases do you have?
What fears do you have?
What judgments do you have?
What narratives do you hold?
What personal experience do you have?
What values do you hold?
What healing potential do you think is possible?

Activity 19: Tracking the Therapeutic Cycle

The therapeutic cycle is a sacred journey from the sterile void of rigid patterns into the fertile void of infinite possibility. Using a recording of a session for this activity is recommended. If that is not possible, recall a recent session.

Awareness: In what ways did you come into presence with your client? How did you come out of presence? How did you follow the client's energy?

Creating a map: What reflections did you offer that were pins on the map of the client's inner world? What did you learn about your client's level of awareness and disruptions to contact?

Identify an inner conflict: What aspects of the client's inner world cause them distress?

Explore distorted life force: Where is energy blocked in the client? What is thwarting the client's alignment?

Set up an experiment: What experiment did you do? What did the client discover about themselves?

Sterile void: Did you pause for raw emotion? Did you make room for the client to feel their own frustration with themselves?

Fertile void: When were moments of catharsis? What old energy did the client mobilize? How did they seem when they discovered new possibilities for themselves?

Activity 20: Facilitating Spiritual Alignment

The client holds within them everything they need to heal, integrate, and come back home to their spiritual alignment. When we honor their innate spirituality as the catalyst for their healing, we create space for their inherent wisdom to process old emotions and complete unresolved experiences. It's the client's wisdom that leads this work, not us. We are simply the mirror and support they need to open to this deep work.

The following process has been designed to support you in facilitating spiritual alignment for your clients. Find a practice partner to explore the following steps. When you are complete, ask them for feedback.

Step 1: Identify and Name

- Once your client shares a feeling or a thought that is causing them distress, have them close their eyes and bring their awareness to this aspect of themselves.
- Invite them to name this aspect of their inner world. For example, if it's a sensation, they might name it fear or protection. If it's a thought, they might name it judgment or self-loathing.
- Reflect back to them the essence of what is being blocked or held in their energy (i.e. the consciousness being held in the sensation, narrative, etc.).

Step 2: Witness

- Now that this aspect has been named, invite the client to wrap it with awareness.
- You might say to them, "Without trying to change this aspect of yourself and without trying to figure it out, allow yourself to be the loving witness. Let this part of you know that you see it."
- You may want to invite them to say to this aspect, "I see you. I see that you are thinking/feeling ...."

Step 3: Validate

- Now that this aspect has been witnessed, invite the client to validate it.
- Invite them to take a few breaths of validation and self-compassion.
- Once their breath seems to have created more spaciousness, invite them to say to themselves, "It makes sense to me that you ...."
  - If this is a thought, have them validate the thought pattern.
- If this is an emotion, have them validate the emotional experience.

Step 4: Give It a Voice

- Now that this aspect has been validated, create an opening for this aspect to be heard.
- If this sensation or thought had a voice, what would it say?
  - With their words, have them vocalize from this aspect of themselves in the first person.
  - For example, if they are tending to tension in their jaw, their jaw might say, "I can't let go."
- If they are tending to a thought pattern, perhaps the mind says, "I need to anticipate in order to stay safe."

Step 5: Be Curious

- Now that this aspect has spoken, be curious about it.
- Invite the client to sit in curiosity by asking them, "Is there anything you want to ask (this aspect of yourself)?"
- Why is it here?
- What does it need from you?
- Allow the answer to come forth naturally.

Step 6: Deepen into Contact

- Now that this aspect has been contacted, invite the client to open to themselves.
- Invite them to give themselves what they need.
- Invite them to breathe in the breath of love and allow their emotions to move through themselves.
- Honor what they have discovered about themselves as they deepen into contact.

Step 7: Self-Responsibility

- From this place of openness, invite them to make a commitment to honor themselves.
- Ask them, "From this place, is there anything you are ready to commit to yourself?"
- Support them in only agreeing to something they are fully ready to embody.
- For example, perhaps this aspect of themselves needed love. Their commitment may be, "I am ready to be gentle with myself."
- Or perhaps this aspect needed to feel safe. Their commitment may be, "I commit to listening to myself and discovering what I need to feel safe."
- If they have a hard time with this step, support them by sharing how you're hearing it. "I am hearing this as, 'I am ready to ….'"

Reference

Kwiker, H. (2023). *Align: Living and loving from the true self.* Mantra Books.

◼ Index

Page numbers in *italics* indicate figures.